Luminaries of the Past
Stories of Fifty Extraordinary Nurses

Written by
Mary Beth Modic and Joyce J. Fitzpatrick
Illustrated by
Sarah K. Turner

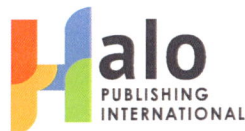

Halo
PUBLISHING
INTERNATIONAL

"Royalties from this book will be used to support future nurse leaders through the Marian K. Shaughnessy Nurse Leadership Academy at the Frances Payne Bolton School of Nursing, Case Western Reserve University."

ISBN: 978-1-61244-920-3
LCCN: 2020919905

Halo
PUBLISHING
INTERNATIONAL

Halo Publishing International, LLC
8000 W Interstate 10, Suite 600
San Antonio, Texas 78230
www.halopublishing.com

Printed and bound in the United States of America

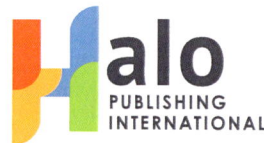

"This new children's book profiling global nurse leaders who changed the world captures historical contributions of diverse nurse leaders from different cultures and background which any child can identify with as a role model. The stories of compassion, triumphant struggles during adversities and perseverance as a change agent in the community are narratives that migrant nurses like myself can relate to and aspire to emulate. What a novel process to illustrate nurses' as superheroes with the personal true stories of 50 exemplary nurses across the globe."

Mary Joy Garcia-Dia, DNP, RN, FAAN
President, 2020-2022
Philippine Nurses Association of America

"It's critically important that the public recognizes the essential role that nurses play. This has been at no time more evident than during the COVID-19 pandemic when nurses, along with others on the healthcare team, are risking their lives to care for patients. We need more nurses using their skills and knowledge to care for patients all over the world."

Suzanne Gordon, co-author of *From Silence to Voice: What Nurses Know and Must Communicate to the Public and author of Life Support: Three Nurses on the Frontlines.*

"What a remarkable collection of biographical sketches of nurses--some well- known in the nursing community and others known well beyond-- and how their work transformed the world, sometimes in unexpected ways. There are too few books to inspire future nurses or to tell our story. This beautiful book is truly a gift."

Carol M. Musil, PhD, RN, FAAN, FGSA
Dean and Edward J. and Louise Mellen Professor
Frances Payne Bolton School of Nursing
Case Western Reserve University

"What a wonderful opportunity this book provides for exploring the depth and character of nursing luminaries whose journey demonstrates how true heroes are made. The authors have included the best and the brightest among us and clearly point out the difference their lives and careers made in the lives of others and in transforming healthcare. This book is a must read for all who celebrate the contribution of women and men who as nurses changed themselves and transformed their world. They serve as a role model for all of us and encourage our own journey and call us to transform healthcare in our own time. This book lifts the spirit and encourages hope in a time of challenge for us all."

Tim Porter-O'Grady, DM, EdD, APRN, FAAN, FACCWS
Senior Partner, Health Systems, TPOG Associates, Tucson, AZ.
Clinical Professor, School of Nursing, Emory University, Atlanta GA.

"Truth is often stranger and more moving than fiction, and that rings true in these stories of 50 nursing luminaries. Nurses are everywhere, in the places where no one else would go, caring for those who everyone else has abandoned. There stories are exciting and guaranteed to move the emotions and imagination of middle-school children, and perhaps propel the most daring into nursing with a life-long passion.

The nurses' heroism as well as their skill in public policy is hard to ignore, whether it is Dix and the development of the first public hospitals for the mentally ill; Nightingale and her worldwide work to reform military health care; Peplau and the development of a scientific base for psychiatric nursing; Christman and his quest for men in nursing; or Whitman and his entry into nursing as a conscientious objector during the Civil War.

This is a work of art and will make a significant addition to the curriculum for middle-school children."

Lucille A. Joel, EdD, APN, FAAN
Distinguished Professor
Rutgers-The State University of New Jersey
School of Nursing
New Brunswick-Newark-Blackwood, New Jersey
Past President, American Nurses Association

"What better way to capture the interest of middle school-age children than a book of exciting short stories about amazing nurse leaders? I can't thank the authors enough for bringing the legacy of these transformational nurses to life. Children, and the public, will gain insight into how nurses make a huge difference to the entire world. A must-read!"

Rosanne Raso DNP, RN, NEA-BC, FAAN, FAONL
VP and Chief Nursing Officer, New York-Presbyterian / Weill Cornell
Editor-in-Chief, Nursing Management, The Journal of Excellence in Nursing Leadership

"This is a truly inspiring book featuring nurse luminaries who made unique contributions to their nursing profession and to society. As a nurse who chose health policy/lobbying as a career, I am proud to help shape legislation that impact patients and their access to innovative medicines. Whether you advocate at the bedside or on Capitol Hill, nurses are instrumental in helping legislators understand how the policies they are voting on can help or harm their constituents (our patients)."

Sharon (Brigner) Lamberton, MS, RN
Deputy Vice President at PhRMA (Pharmaceutical Research and Manufacturers of America)
Past President National Student Nurses Association 1996-97

"Luminaries of the past is a beautiful book telling the treasured stories of nurses who are the foundation of our profession. Thank you Joyce and Mary Beth."

Eunice Cole,
ANA Past President (1982-1986)

This book is dedicated to the future nurses of the world who, like the individuals who came before them, will reduce suffering, promote health and well-being, and advocate for social justice.

Contents

Note regarding the use of the prefix "Nurse" in text:

Several of the nurses have earned doctorates, e.g., PhD and EdD degrees. Rather than referring to them as "Drs.," which might confuse them with medical doctors, we have chosen to refer to them as "Nurses."

INTRODUCTION

Nurses work in hospitals, clinics, and schools. They work on cruise ships and at summer camps, and they debate in the United States Congress. They are scientists, inventors, and authors. They care for newborns when they take their first breath and the dying when they take their last. Nurses work everywhere, yet they remain invisible, much of their work unknown to the public.

This book was written to celebrate the contributions of 50 remarkable nurses who made a difference in the world. They fought for better care of the sick and better health-care for all. They revolutionized the way nurses were educated. They campaigned for racial, gender, and social justice. Their work collectively saved millions of lives.

There are more than 27 million nurses in the world today who carry on the work of these noteworthy nurses.

Note regarding the image on the front cover:

The Nightingale Lamp is pictured on the front cover. It is a replica of the lamp that Nightingale carried while nursing the wounded during the Crimean War. This replica was found in a souk in Istanbul, Turkey. Artists often fictionalized the Nightingale Lamp and pictured her with an Aladdin lamp rather than the lamp pictured here.

Cover idea: Joselyn Modic Banda

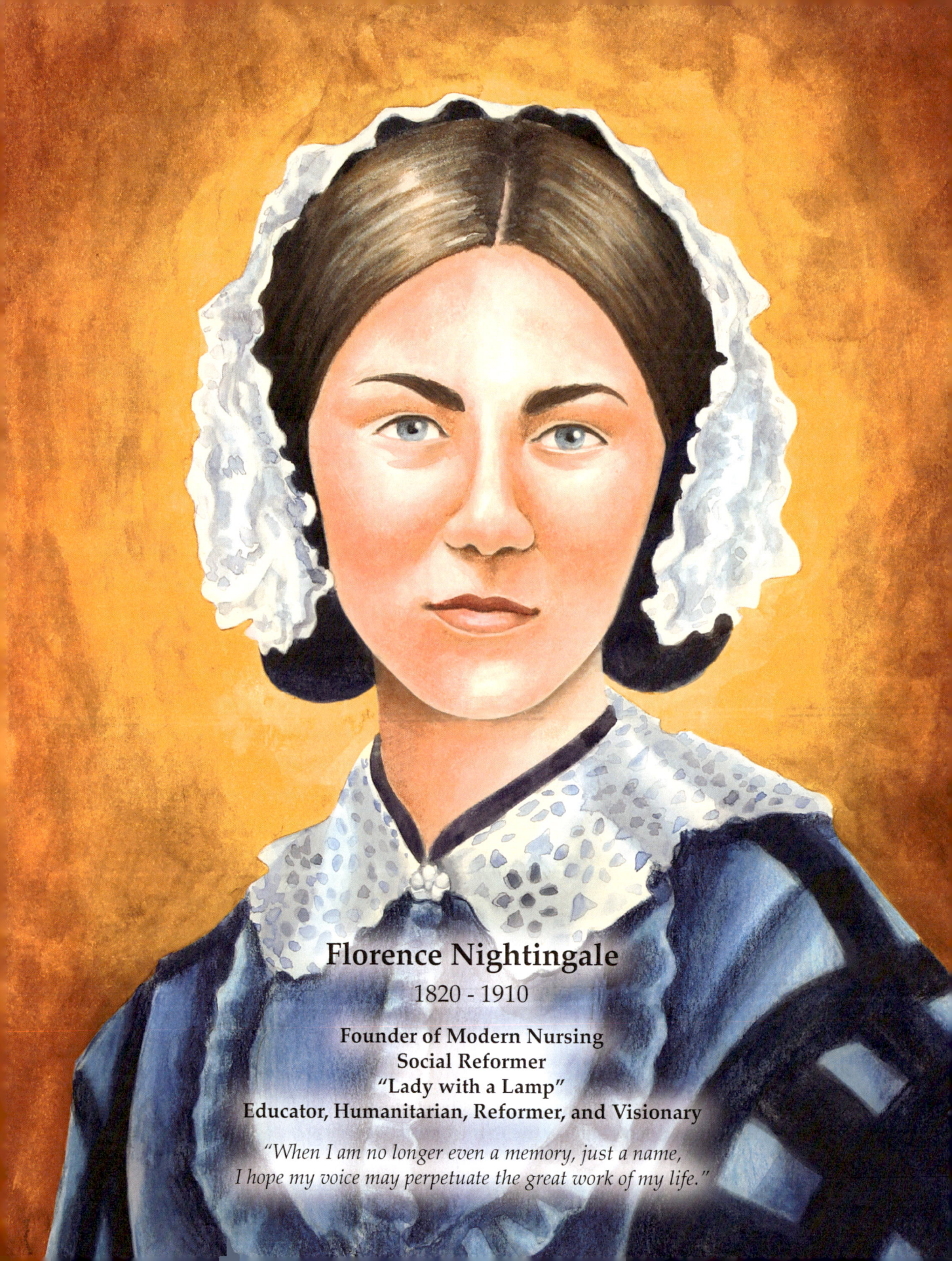

Florence Nightingale

1820 - 1910

Founder of Modern Nursing
Social Reformer
"Lady with a Lamp"
Educator, Humanitarian, Reformer, and Visionary

"When I am no longer even a memory, just a name,
I hope my voice may perpetuate the great work of my life."

Florence Nightingale was born on May 12, 1820, to William Edward and Frances (Franny) Smith Nightingale in Florence, Italy, and was named after the city of her birth. Her older sister, Frances Parthenope, was also named after the city in which she was born. Parthenope, a Greek settlement in Italy, is now a part of Naples, Italy. The family moved back to England when Florence was just 1 year old. Florence's family was British and wealthy, and they traveled frequently throughout Europe. Florence's father had inherited a vast fortune from his uncle, which allowed the family to spend time at their 2 estates. Florence and Parthe were taught by their Cambridge University-educated father, who held progressive ideas about women's education. The two girls received instruction in history, philosophy, classical literature, and mathematics. Florence became fluent in French, German, Italian, and Turkish. The Nightingale family had many prominent house guests, so Parthe and Florence were surrounded by influential thinkers, politicians, leaders, and educators of the time. Florence learned to ask questions, defend her thinking, and gain the respect of men in power.

In 1837, Florence was 17 years old. She believed God had called her to live a life of service, relieving the pain and suffering of others. She knew that becoming a nurse would be the answer to God's "divine call." Florence's parents were not happy that she wished to become a nurse, as the work was not acceptable for a woman of Florence's social status. Through her family travels and connections, Florence met an English-born Parisian hostess named Mary Clarke. Florence bonded with "Clarkey," who was an outspoken woman who demonstrated that women could be equal to men. Although there was a 27-year age difference between them, Clarkey was one of Florence's closest friends, and she influenced Florence's life and thinking for 40 years.

Florence received an education reserved only for boys, as girls were expected to marry young, raise children, and spend most of their time in domestic routines. Florence could not imagine living this kind of life, although she had received several marriage proposals. For 7 years, Richard Monckton Milnes, a poet and politician, courted Florence. She thought he was a smart man and hoped that he would accept a "working wife," but he could not. After Florence refused Richard's marriage proposal, Richard married another woman, but Florence and Richard remained life-long friends.

In 1849, Florence's parents approved of her plans to accompany Charles and Selina Bracebridges, family friends of the Nightingales, to visit Egypt, Greece, and Europe. The Bracebridges never had children but treated Florence like a daughter. The Bracebridges loved to travel and were delighted to have Florence travel with them, as they had some health concerns and knew that they could rely on Florence to take care of them should they become ill. Her mother, disappointed that Florence had turned down a marriage proposal, thought the trip would be good for her. This trip would prove life altering for Florence.

The final stop on her trip, before returning to England, was a visit to the Kaiserwerth Institute of Protestant Deaconesses in Dusseldorf, Germany. Unbeknownst to her parents, Mrs. Bracebridges had made arrangements for Florence to meet Pastor Theodor Fliedner, the founder of the German training school for nurses. For two weeks, Florence was able to observe the operations of the school.

An important person who helped Florence develop the case she would use to convince her family that nursing was her destiny was Doctor Elizabeth Blackwell. Elizabeth Blackwell was the first woman doctor in the United States. The Bracebridges introduced Florence to Elizabeth, who served as a role model. The two shared similar ideas about politics, philosophy, and the potential contributions of women. They spent many hours in conversation about the future of medicine and nursing.

Society viewed nursing as work that required little skill and knowledge, and it certainly did not make one wealthy. Florence's family learned of her secret visit to Kaiserwerth, and her mother and Parthe were angry. To escape the emotional intensity of her home, Florence accepted invitations to care for elderly family members. This opportunity reinforced her desire to become a nurse. Her father, who was always proud of his "misfit" daughter, finally gave his approval for her to study nursing. On July 6, 1851, at the age of 31, Florence began her 3-month training at Kaiswerwerth. After completing her education, she went to Paris to receive additional nursing training from the Sisters of Mercy.

Following her schooling, in 1853, Nurse Nightingale became the superintendent of the Institution for the Care of Sick Gentlewomen in Distressed Circumstances in London, which was a 27-bed hospital with 3 floors. Florence had many gifts. She was intelligent, hardworking, and determined. Perhaps her greatest talent was her ability to lead others.

In 1854, a terrible illness was overtaking the people of London. Over 500 people died in 10 days. The number of deaths would have been greater had the residents not fled the neighborhood where the outbreak occurred. Florence became superintendent at the Middlesex Hospital, where hundreds of Londoners, sick with the life-threatening illness, came for care at all hours of the day and night. Florence worked with Doctor John Snow. He identified the source of the illness as the water pump on Broad Street. The illness was cholera, a bacterial infection that affects the small intestine and causes diarrhea and dehydration. If not treated quickly, the infected person can die. The lives of Londoners were saved when the local government removed the handle on the water pump so no one could drink the water.

From a young age, Florence demonstrated that she was a kind and caring person. While traveling in Athens, Greece, with the Bracebridges, Florence rescued an owlet from a group of children who were bothering it. She named the owlet Athena, after the place where she found it, and often carried it in her pocket. Florence enjoyed Athena's companionship for 5 years until the Crimean War broke out.

March of 1854, Great Britain entered the Crimean War to fight beside France, Turkey, and Sardinia against the Russians, who were trying to expand into what is known today as Romania. Sidney Herbert, the Secretary of War, wrote to Nurse Nightingale and urged her to organize a group of nurses to sail to Crimea (now Istanbul, Turkey) to help with the increasingly devastating conditions of the hospitals, especially at Scutari.

Florence recruited 38 women volunteer nurses she had trained, along with 15 Catholic nuns, to join her in the plan to assist in the military hospital. They found the wounded soldiers lying in blood-soaked sheets, their hygiene neglected, and rats running through the wards. Food was served raw or overcooked, and the staff had to walk 3-4 miles to deliver it. Florence began using a piece of chalk to number each cot, and she kept detailed notes about each patient's illness as well as recovery or cause of death. The nurses bathed and cleaned the soldiers, applied fresh bandages, wrapped them in blankets, and provided nutritious meals. Florence demanded that the soldiers be treated according to their clinical condition, not their rank.

During her first winter in the war hospital in Scutari, Nurse Nightingale noted that ten times more soldiers died from the illnesses caused by infection and neglect than from battle wounds. She demanded that the British government send workers from the Department of Sanitation. The death rate decreased dramatically after the changes she proposed were put into place. She believed that mental health was important to health and healing. She helped soldiers write letters to their loved ones and read the letters they received. She walked the halls at night, carrying a small lamp, tending to patients. Thus, she was named "The Lady with the Lamp" by the soldiers.

After the war ended, Florence returned to England a hero. Queen Victoria of England presented Florence with a brooch called the "Nightingale Jewel." The brooch was created by Prince Albert to recognize Florence's extraordinary service to her country, as there were no medals suitable for women civilians at the time. She also received a donation of $250,000 from the government, which she used to fund the Saint Thomas Hospital and Nightingale Training School for Nurses.

After her experiences in the hospital in Scutari during the Crimean War, she made the design and care in hospitals a major focus in her writings as well as in her ideas for health reform in peace and conflict. She spent the next several years teaching others about proper hospital care.

Among Florence's most significant contributions were sanitary reforms and statistics. She brought changes in sanitary conditions to the military hospitals. She pointed out that contaminated water, poor ventilation, and overcrowding led to poor health outcomes and even death among the sick soldiers. She was a true pioneer in the graphic presentation of statistics, developing a form of the "pie chart" called a "coxcomb," which she used to describe the seasonal changes in deaths in the military field hospitals. She was the first woman inducted into the Royal Statistical Society in 1858.

Through the many books and more than 14,000 letters she wrote, Nightingale influenced the thinking and actions of policy makers in the British government and beyond. She used her connections through friends of her family to influence change in the government and to make sure that better hospital care would be provided in the future. Her works were instrumental in the foundation of the International Red Cross and the United Nations.

Nightingale is best known for two things: her nursing of soldiers during the Crimean War and for being the founder of modern nursing. She created the first schools of nursing to prepare women to care for the sick. When Nightingale started out, there was no such thing as nursing in the way that we know nurses and nursing today. Hospitals were places of the last resort, not places where the sick could be returned to health. Nightingale taught nurses to care for the sick and to introduce natural therapies that would lead to health, such as clean air, healthy food, and clean bedding, and she taught the nurses the scientific reasons for their care. Further, she set an example of compassion and commitment to patient care that continue to be the foundations of nursing today.

The Nightingale School for Nurses that she founded in 1860 is now called the Florence Nightingale Faculty of Nursing and Midwifery at King's College London. There are two Florence Nightingale museums, one in London and one at the military barracks in Istanbul, Turkey. Her birthday, May 12, is celebrated yearly as International Nurses Day. The year 2020 was declared the Year of the Nurse and Midwife by the World Health Organization in honor of the 200th anniversary of her birth.

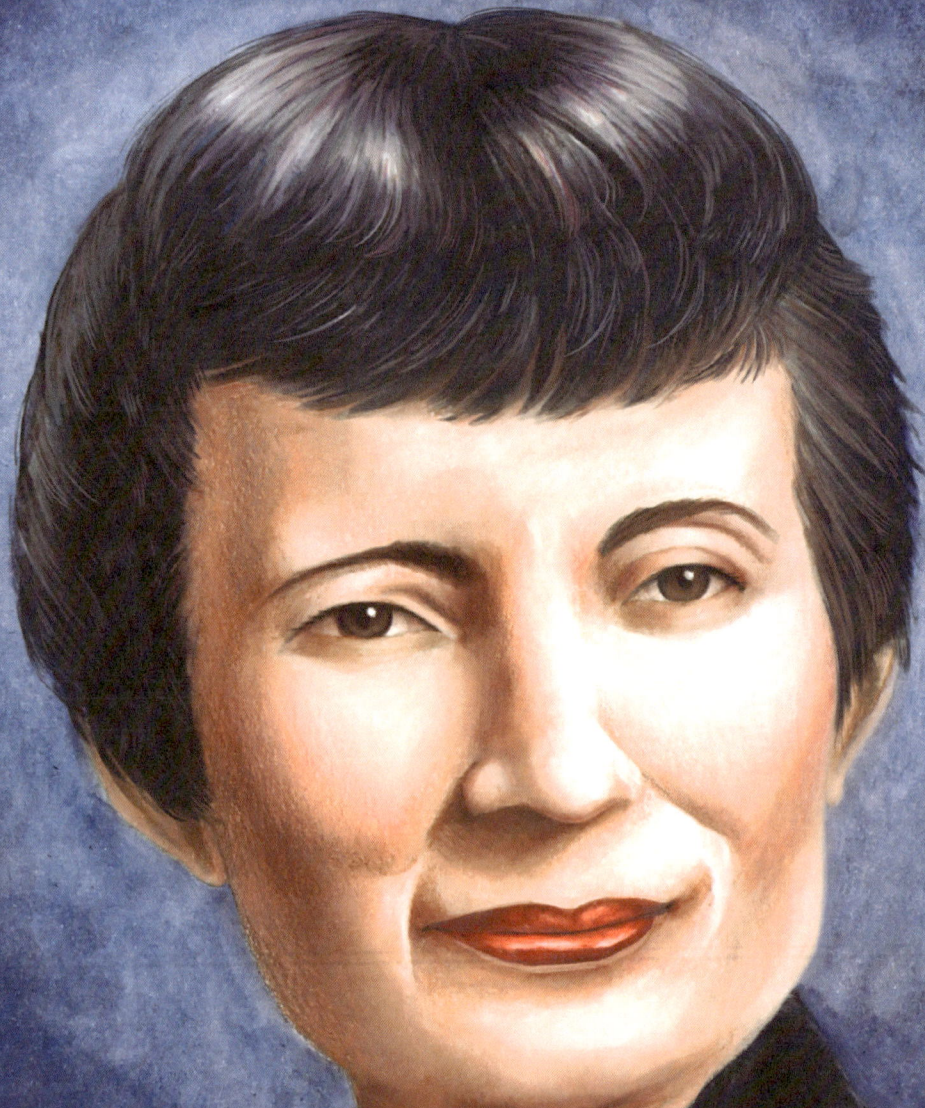

Faye Abdellah

1919 – 2017

Deputy Surgeon General
Rear Admiral, Federal Nursing Services
Pioneer in Nursing Research
Educator, Pioneer, and Visionary

"We cannot wait for the world to change . . . Those of us with intelligence, purpose, and vision must take the lead and change the world . . . I promise never to rest until my work has been completed!"

Faye Glenn Abdellah was born in New York City on March 13, 1919, to H. B. and Margaret Glenn Abdellah. She had one older brother, Marty. May 6, 1937, was the day that Faye decided to become a nurse. It was the day that the Hindenburg, a German airbus, caught fire and exploded, killing 35 of the 97 people aboard. Faye and her brother went to the aid of the victims.

Faye received her initial nursing preparation from Fitkin Memorial Hospital (Ann May School of Nursing) in New Jersey. This was followed by a liberal arts and chemistry degree from Rutgers University. Her nursing education was advanced through Teachers College, Columbia University. There, she received three degrees: a BS, a Master of Arts, and a PhD in educational psychology.

From 1945 to 1949, Nurse Abdellah was a professor of nursing arts, pharmacology, and medical nursing at Yale University School of Nursing. Early in her career, while on the faculty of Yale University, she became frustrated by the lack of scientific basis in the National League of Nursing guidelines, and she proceeded to burn a stack of the curriculum guides in the Yale courtyard. She often mentioned, with some humor, that it took well over a year for her to pay for the books she destroyed.

From 1950 to 1954, she served in active duty during the Korean War. She earned the distinguished ranking equivalent to a Navy Rear Admiral. She was the highest ranked woman and nurse in the Federal Nursing Services at the time. Faye was the first nurse officer to earn the ranking of a two-star rear admiral.

In 1981, she was appointed as deputy to Surgeon General C. Everett Koop. Faye was the first nurse and the first woman to serve as a Deputy Surgeon General of the United States. She worked to influence health care policy and educate the public about HIV-AIDS, hospice care, substance abuse, and smoking and alcoholism. She served in this position until 1989, when she became dean of a new graduate school of nursing and the first federal school of nursing, which was the Uniformed Services University of the Health Sciences. Faye built the faculty and student body of this new school and prepared thousands of nurse clinicians and researchers to serve in the US military ranks.

Nurse Abdellah was a pioneer in nursing science and research. She developed a model of nursing that she labeled "Twenty-One Nursing Problems." The 21-problem list included physical, sociological, and emotional needs of patients. Her model of nursing was radical at the time of initial development, as she was one of the first nurses to advocate for nurses to diagnose health problems as part of their professional role. Her model of nursing is still used to teach nurses today.

One of her many pioneering accomplishments was the creation of the National Institute of Nursing Research (NINR) at the National Institutes of Health. Before this time, there was no federal organization dedicated to nursing research. Elected officials did not think that nurses needed to conduct research or that they could use discoveries in medical science to care for patients and the public. Faye rallied nurse scientists throughout the U.S. to accomplish this monumental task. She subsequently was instrumental in creating the Friends of the NINR.

Throughout her career Nurse Faye Glenn Abdellah received more than 10 honorary doctorates from U.S. universities. She used her intellect, curiosity, and extraordinary leadership skills to set a new standard for nursing practice. Faye, like Florence Nightingale many years before her, cleared a path for women and nurse researchers in society.

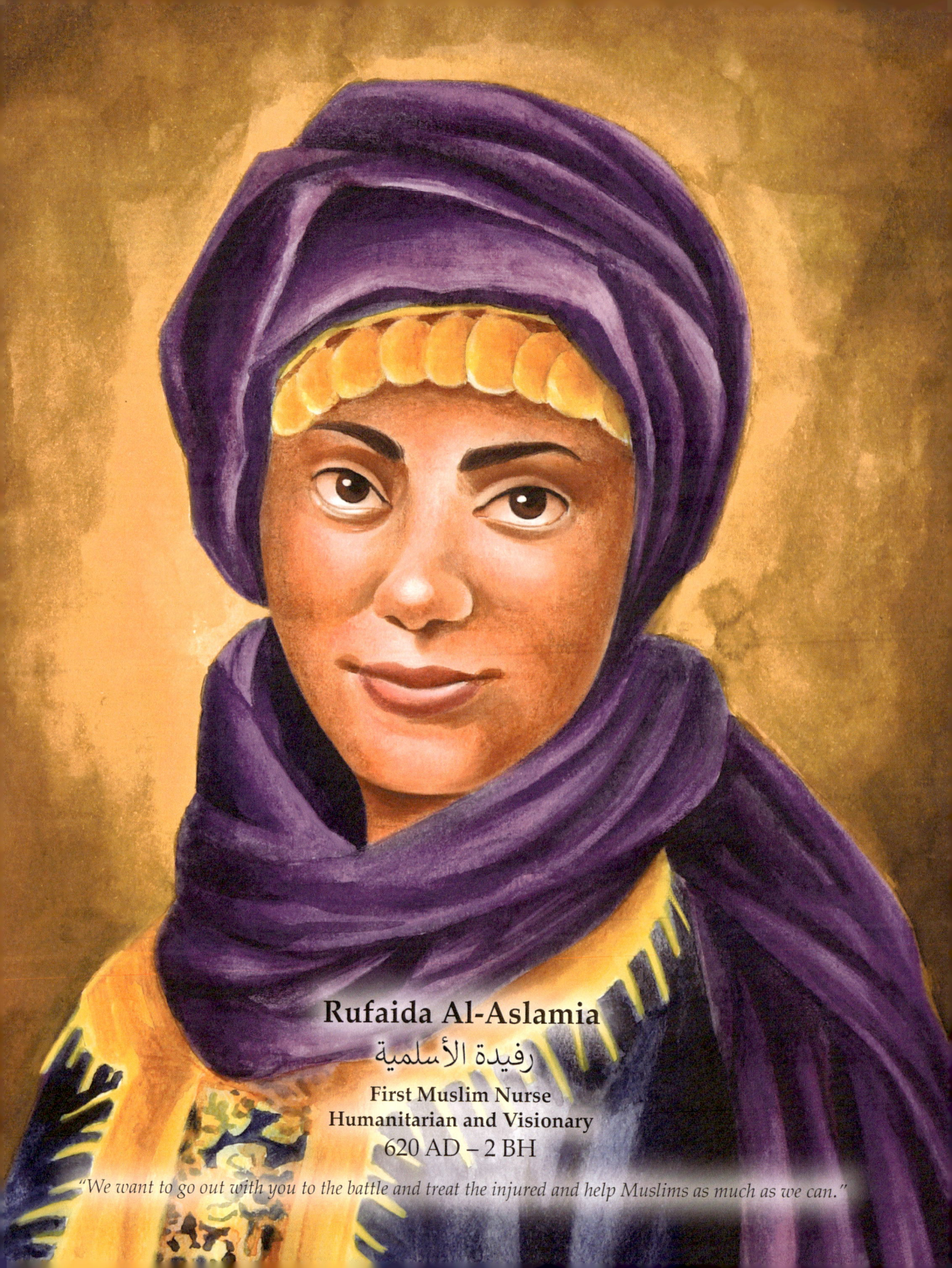

Rufaida Al-Aslamia

رفيدة الأسلمية

First Muslim Nurse
Humanitarian and Visionary
620 AD – 2 BH

"We want to go out with you to the battle and treat the injured and help Muslims as much as we can."

Rufaida Al-Aslamiyah was thought to be born in the year 620 in the ancient city of Yathrib (now called Madinah) in Saudi Arabia. Much of what is known about Rufaida and her life is based upon stories that have been passed down through the generations. Her name can be spelled differently based on the translation that is used. Little is known about Rufaida's mother. Her father was a doctor, and Rufaida learned the practice of medicine from him. She used her knowledge, compassion, and organizational skills to care for the wounded soldiers on the battlefield. Rufaida is known as the first Muslim nurse in history.

Rufaida was one of the first people in Madinah to accept Islam and welcome the holy prophet Muhammad (PBUH) into her city. The initials "PBUH" are often used after Muhammad's name and mean "peace be upon him." Muhammad was a deeply spiritual man and was the founder of Islam. Muhammad began receiving revelations from Allah when he was 40 years of age and began sharing the messages with his tribe. He endured a great deal of hardships while spreading the word of Allah. By the year 630, Mohammad had united most of Arabia under a single religion. The revelations he shared were collected and became the basis for the Quran.

Rufaida practiced nursing during the holy wars. During this time in Islam, the female nurse was called "Al-Assiyah," from the word "assaa," which translates to "curing the wounds." Rufaida believed that she had the opportunity to express her faith by nursing the soldiers on the battlefield. She recruited women to assist her in this work. The women, known as "companions," fed the soldiers, provided water to quench their thirst, and provided shelter to protect the soldiers from the intense heat and wind of the desert. Her reputation as an excellent nurse became well known, and during several intense battles, Muhammad directed the casualties to her tent.

After the wars were over, Muhammad gave Rufaida permission to erect a tent within his mosque. This allowed Rufaida to continue her work as a nurse by providing care and health education to members of her community. She cared for the poor, the orphaned, and the handicapped, advocating for their well-being. Rufaida established the first school of nursing and is believed to have created the first code of ethics for nursing.

Because of Rufaida Al-Asalamia's work, her dedication to her faith, and her devotion to the sick, nursing is considered an honorable career for Muslim women in keeping with the Islamic tradition. In Pakistan, she is honored with a building named after her at the Aga Khan University School of Nursing. The Rufaida Al-Aslamia Prize is awarded annually to a nursing student who provides exceptional nursing care to patients. The recipient is determined by members of the medical staff at the University of Bahrain.

While Florence Nightingale is known as the founder of modern nursing, it is Rufaida Al-Aslamia who practiced the art of nursing in the Muslim world 1,200 years earlier, which is a fact that scholars of Muslim nursing want the world to know.

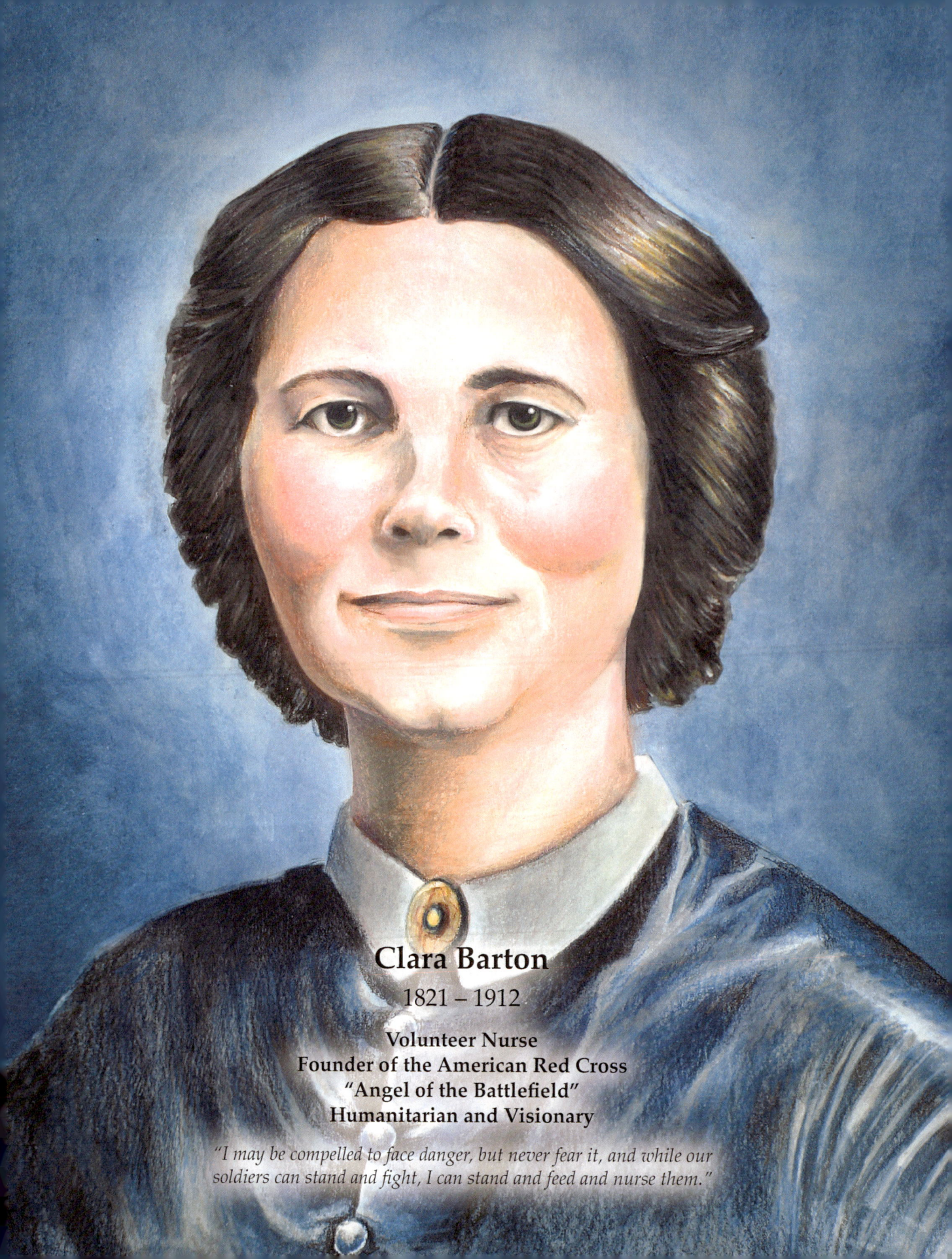

Clara Barton

1821 – 1912

Volunteer Nurse
Founder of the American Red Cross
"Angel of the Battlefield"
Humanitarian and Visionary

"I may be compelled to face danger, but never fear it, and while our
soldiers can stand and fight, I can stand and feed and nurse them."

Clarissa "Clara" Harlowe Barton was born on December 25, 1821, in Oxford, Massachusetts. Clara had four older siblings, and her father was a farmer. When she was 12 years old, she took care of her brother David, who became injured in a barn-raising accident, and nursed him back to health. This event began her life of service to those in need.

Her parents encouraged her to become a teacher, and eventually she opened a school for the children of mill workers. She had a gift for teaching and was able to keep even the rowdiest children engaged in learning. She moved to New Jersey and opened the first free school in the area. She resigned from teaching at the school after learning a male colleague was getting paid more than she. She was a true feminist and did not believe that women should get paid less than men for doing the same job!

She moved to Washington, D.C., and worked in the U.S. Patent Office. This job was important because Clara was paid the same salary as a man, and working as a clerk in the U.S. Patent Office, she was able to award inventors a patent. A patent is a property right, and it prevents other inventors from taking ideas or inventions and using it as their own idea. She worked in the government office under President Pierce, President Buchanan, and President Lincoln.

The American Civil War began in 1861, and Clara dedicated herself to helping with the war effort. In 1862, she received official permission to deliver supplies to soldiers on various major battlefields. She was passionate about making sure that the men fighting the war had what they needed. She developed a passion for aiding those in need during disasters and wars. She was known as the "Angel of the Battlefield."

After the war, there were thousands of men whose families did not know what had happened to them. To help their families find them, Clara created the Bureau of Records of Missing Army Men. She published the names of the missing men by state for 4 years and was able to find over 22,000 soldiers both dead and alive. She also made sure that over 13,000 soldiers who died at the Andersonville Prison in Georgia received a proper burial.

While traveling in Europe, Clara learned of the International Red Cross, which was founded in 1864 in Geneva, Switzerland. Clara learned how great of an impact the International Red Cross had and wanted the United States to have something similar. She knew the American Red Cross could participate and positively impact national and global relief efforts for disaster and crisis events.

In 1881, at the age of 60, through writing, teaching, and lobbying, she set up the American Red Cross and served as the first President of the American Red Cross for 23 years. Her vision has resulted in millions of people receiving help and shelter during disasters, safe blood donations, and instruction in first aid.

In 1904, she created the National First Aid Association of America, which aimed to teach people how to take care of themselves and others during accidents and emergencies. She remained passionate about women's rights her whole life and was an advocate for self-education and preparedness for life events. Clara Barton's determination and dedication to helping those in need—regardless of their nationality, race, gender, or belief system—is a lesson for humanity that stands the test of time

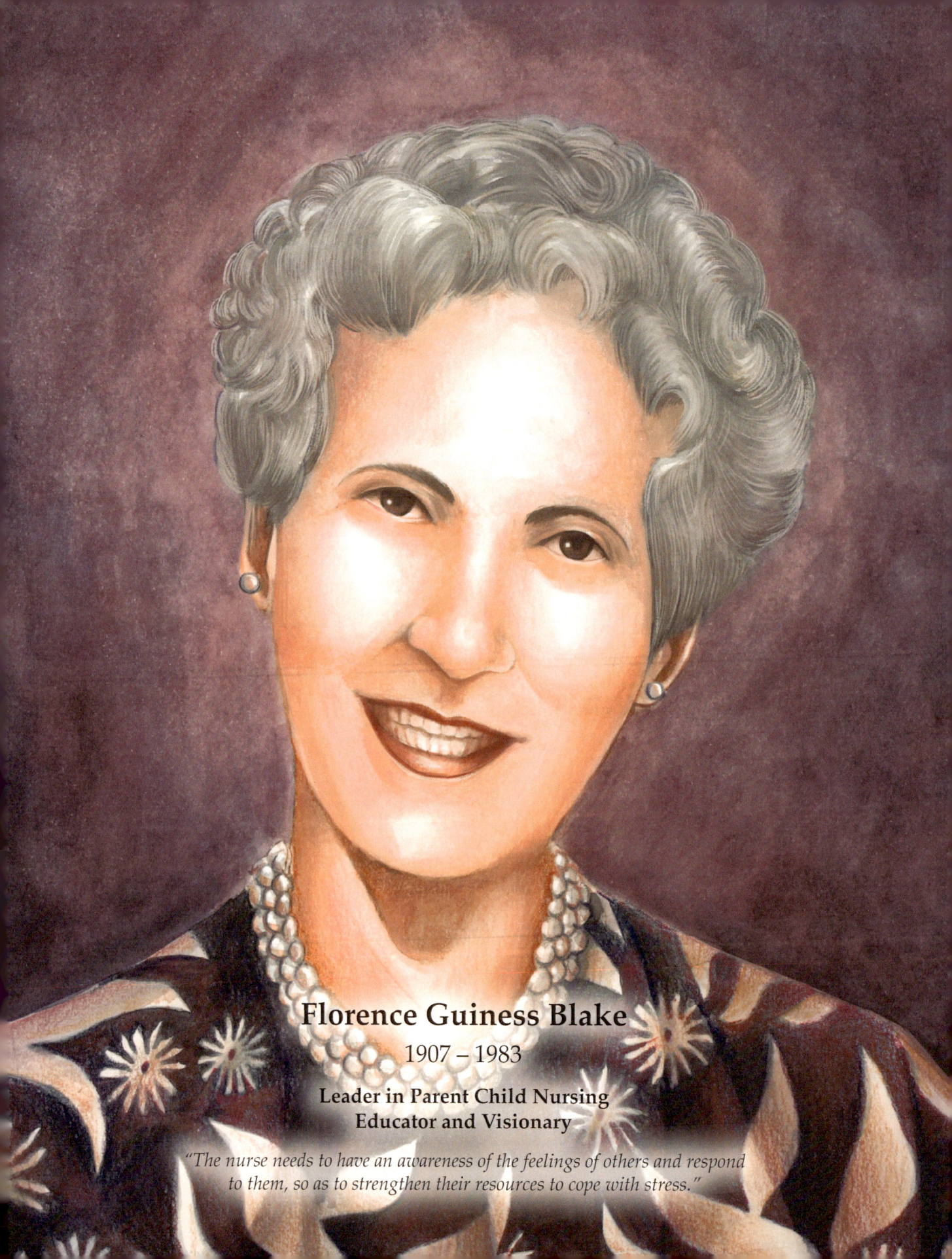

Florence Guiness Blake

1907 – 1983

**Leader in Parent Child Nursing
Educator and Visionary**

*"The nurse needs to have an awareness of the feelings of others and respond
to them, so as to strengthen their resources to cope with stress."*

Florence Guiness Blake was born on November 30, 1907, in Stevens Point, Wisconsin, to Thelma Dunlap and James Blake. Her mother was a musician, and her father was an Episcopalian minister who served in the Belgian Congo. Florence learned the joy of service at an early age, as she and her sister often accompanied their father on home visits. She observed his kindness as he listened and prayed with his homebound parishioners. Her decision to become a nurse was influenced by her father's compassion. Her uncle, a surgeon, encouraged her to attend the Michael Reese School of Nursing, from which she graduated from in 1928.

Florence was recognized by the director of the school as an outstanding student and one who could become an exceptional nursing instructor. She arranged for Florence to spend 3 months at the University of Chicago to learn about supervising and teaching students. After graduation, she taught at the Michael Reese School of Nursing and at Teachers College, Columbia University. After teaching for several years, she returned to the hospital and began caring for sick children. She soon realized that this would be her life's work: to become a pediatric nurse. The word "pediatric" means "healer of children." She also taught in nursery schools to become familiar with how children grow and develop. Florence met nursing faculty from China while she was a student at Teachers College, and they encouraged her to apply for a Rockefeller Grant to teach in Peiping (now Beijing), China. She spent three years in China reflecting on the best way to educate nursing students in pediatric nursing. Before returning to the United States, Nurse Blake spent time observing nursing care of children in different parts of the world.

Upon her return to the United States, Florence enrolled in the master's program at the University of Michigan and graduated in 1941. She taught pediatric nursing at several nursing schools. While at Yale, she worked with child psychiatrist Edith Jackson to promote the benefits of "rooming-in". It was common practice in the 1940s to keep newborns in the nursery "away from their mothers" so that they would not be exposed to infectious diseases. Both Doctor Jackson and Nurse Blake believed that keeping babies in the room with their mothers allowed the baby and mother to bond easily. The baby cried less and breastfed more easily, and the mom had more confidence in caring for her baby.

In 1946, Nurse Blake was invited to design a program of advanced nursing in pediatric nursing at the University of Chicago. She also contributed to various editions of two nursing textbooks. In 1954, Florence wrote the book *The Child, His Parents and the Nurse*. This book was one of the first of its kind to describe how children and their families respond emotionally to illness and how the nurse can be of the most help. It also promoted the importance of involving the parents in the care of the child, which is the standard of care for children today.

Nurse Blake taught at the University of Chicago from 1946 to 1959, until the university closed its nursing program. She studied the needs of critically ill children undergoing open heart surgery and their response to hospitalization.

In 1963, Florence was invited to join the faculty of the University of Wisconsin Madison School of Nursing as the director of the graduate program in nursing. She was a memorable teacher who focused on clinical knowledge in graduate school programs rather than teaching and administration activities. Her visionary work influenced the thinking of doctors as well as nurses.

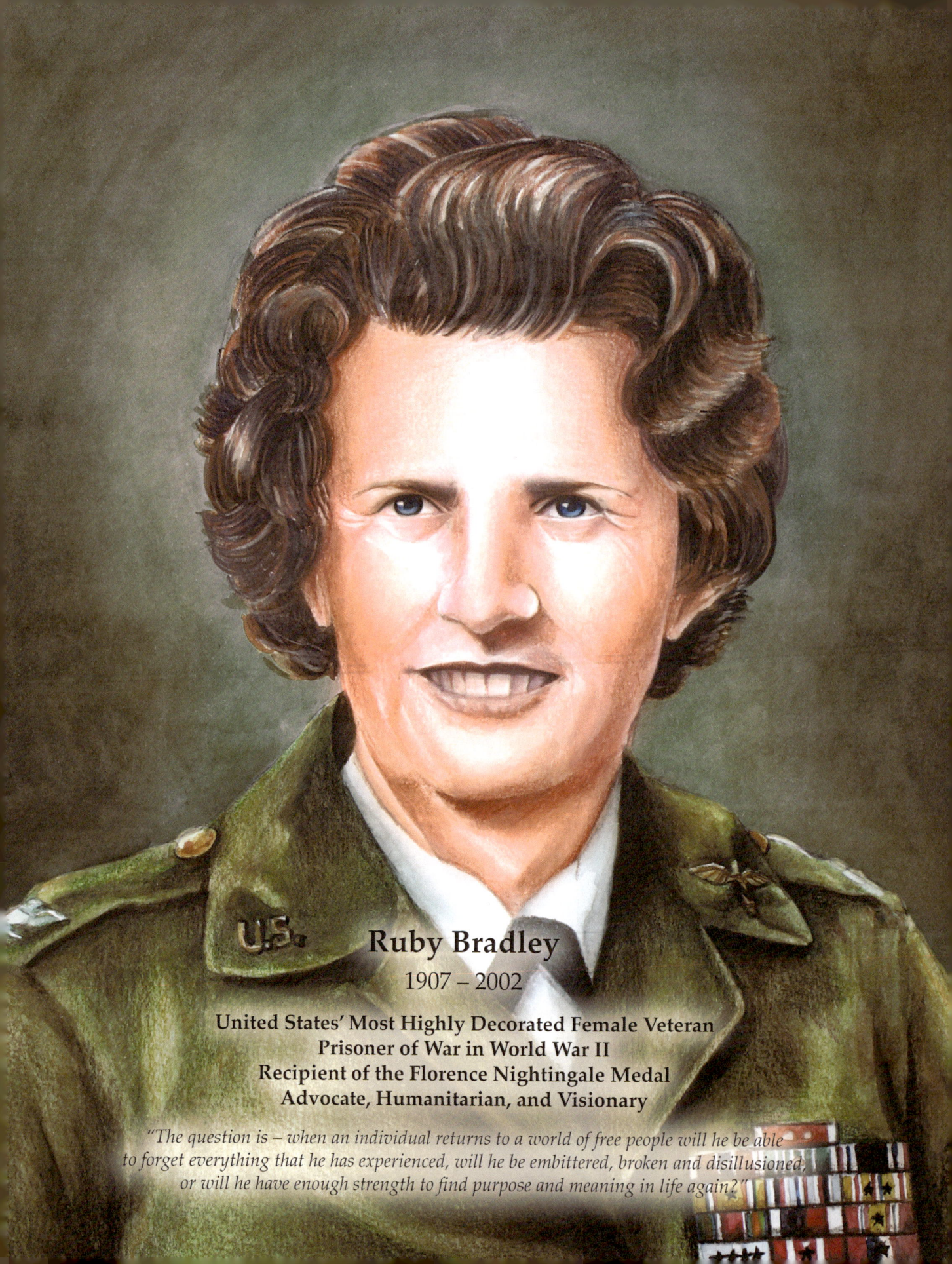

Ruby Bradley

1907 – 2002

**United States' Most Highly Decorated Female Veteran
Prisoner of War in World War II
Recipient of the Florence Nightingale Medal
Advocate, Humanitarian, and Visionary**

*"The question is – when an individual returns to a world of free people will he be able
to forget everything that he has experienced, will he be embittered, broken and disillusioned,
or will he have enough strength to find purpose and meaning in life again?"*

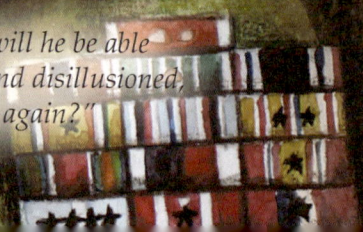

Ruby Grace Bradley was born on a farm on December 19, 1907, in Spencer, West Virginia. She grew up with her parents, Bertha Lynch and Fredrick Bradley, and three siblings. In 1926, there were very few jobs for women, so Ruby enrolled at Glenville Teachers College and became a teacher. Ruby taught in one-room schools in Spencer for four years, and while she loved teaching, she had a longing to see the world and to live a life of adventure. Sally, her younger sister, was a nurse and invited Ruby to Walter Reed Hospital. That experience changed her life. She knew then that nursing was the career for her.

She graduated from Philadelphia General School of Nursing and began working at Walter Reed Hospital. Upon joining the Army Nurse Corps as a surgical nurse, Ruby was told she would never see war by the recruiter. Seven years later, she was transferred to the Philippines, where she served as head nurse at Camp John Hay. Three weeks after the bombing of Pearl Harbor on December 7, 1941, Ruby was captured by the Japanese soldiers. She spent three years as a Prisoner of War (POW).

Ruby and the other captives were sent to Santo Tomas Internment Camp in Manila.

Ruby, a doctor, and a dentist were transported to their old hospital to retrieve toilet tissue by the Japanese guards. They were threatened that only toilet tissue was to be collected and brought back to camp. Under the watchful eyes of their Japanese captors, the trio smuggled medications, surgical instruments, and supplies. They knew they had to risk their lives to bring the supplies back to the camp so that they could treat the sick and wounded prisoners. Ruby assisted in 230 major surgeries and delivered 13 babies while imprisoned. Ruby and the other nurses became creative when their smuggled supplies ran out. Bandages were made out of old bed sheets, and sutures were made out of hemp leaves that were pulled into threads. All of the handmade items and surgical instruments were sterilized by boiling them on a stove. Toys were made for the children by using the stuffing from their mattresses.

The conditions of the camp were horrific. Four out of every 10 American prisoners died of starvation, illness, or abuse. Each prisoner was given a cup of rice to eat. Nurse Bradley would save and ration her rice so that she could feed the starving children. By the time the camp was liberated in February of 1945, Ruby weighed just 86 pounds.

Following World War II, Ruby returned to the United States and earned a baccalaureate degree in nursing education from the University of California in 1949. Once the Korean War broke out, Ruby served as the 8th Army's chief nurse, working to evacuate soldiers on the front lines. Ruby exemplified her commitment to the Nurses' Professional Code of Ethics by never abandoning a patient. She is remembered as the last person on the plane in Pyongyang, North Korea, as her ambulance exploded and the plane was surrounded by 100,000 Chinese soldiers.

Ruby never married, and she retired from the Army at the age of 56. She spent her years in retirement managing a private-duty nursing service in West Virginia.

Colonel Ruby Bradley was the third woman in the Army to be promoted to the rank of colonel in 1968. She was awarded 34 medals and citations of bravery. She was the recipient of the Florence Nightingale Medal, which was bestowed by the Red Cross. Colonel Bradley elevated the practice of nursing in wartime, and when asked about her remarkable career, she responded, "It was all in a day's work."

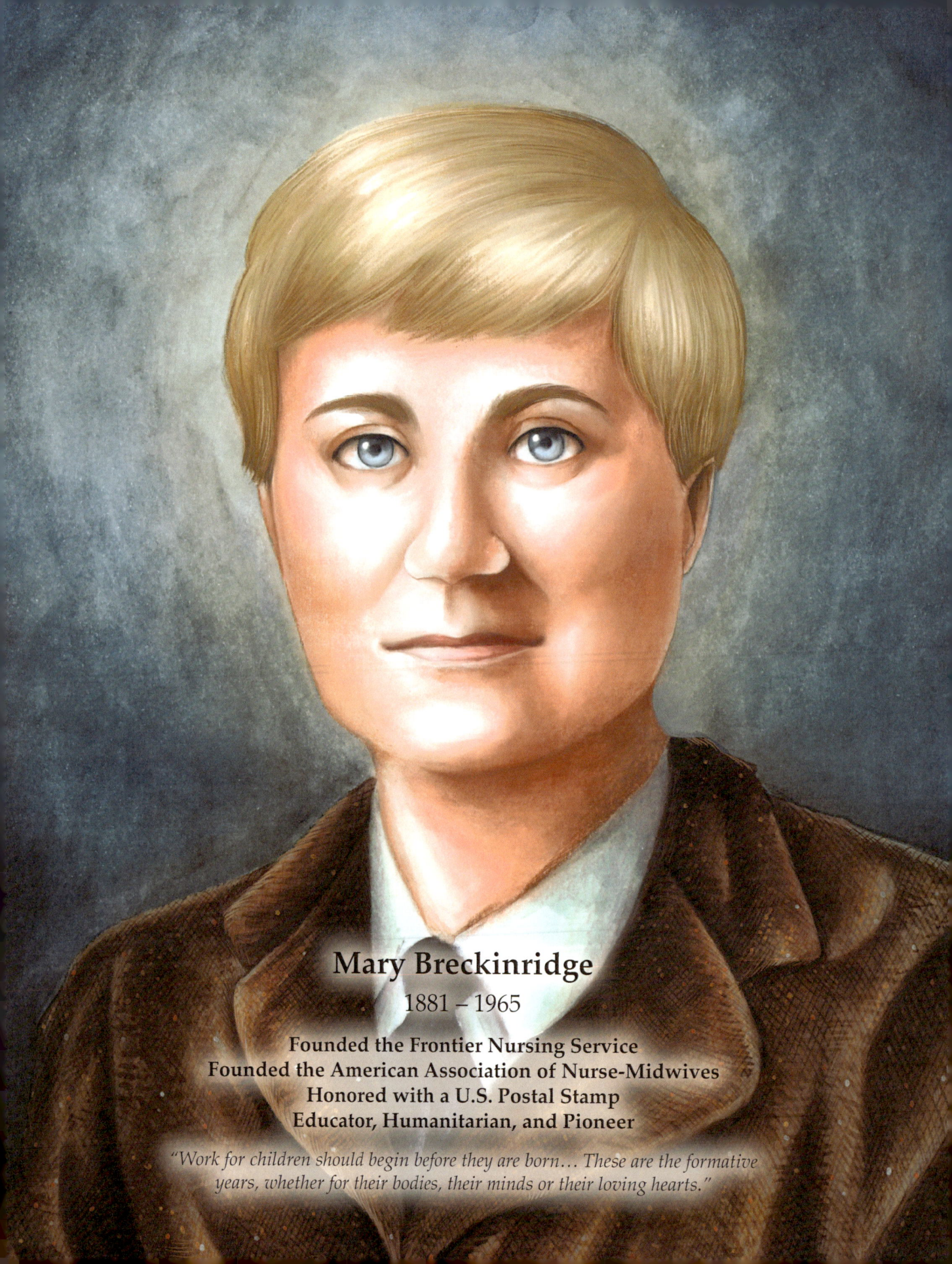

Mary Breckinridge

1881 – 1965

Founded the Frontier Nursing Service
Founded the American Association of Nurse-Midwives
Honored with a U.S. Postal Stamp
Educator, Humanitarian, and Pioneer

"Work for children should begin before they are born… These are the formative years, whether for their bodies, their minds or their loving hearts."

Mary Breckinridge was born in Memphis, Tennessee, on February 17, 1881. She grew up in Washington, D.C., where her father was an Arkansas congressman, and in St. Petersburg, Russia, where her father served as the United States minister to Russia. She also was the granddaughter of United States Vice President John C. Breckinridge. She was educated in private boarding schools in Lausanne, Switzerland, and Stamford, Connecticut. Mary was introduced to nursing when she was 14 years old and learned that her brother was delivered by a Russian nurse midwife. This experience was very influential in Mary's dream to bring the practice of nurse midwifery to the United States and the creation of the Frontier Nursing Service.

Mary enjoyed the outdoors and was a skilled hunter and horsewoman. She valued her independence and had the financial means to remain single, but she chose to marry. The marriage ended after two years, as her husband died unexpectedly. Following his death, she entered St. Luke's Hospital School of Nursing in New York City and graduated in 1910. She returned to Arkansas and taught French and hygiene at a women's school where she met and married her second husband, the president of the school. She had two children, both of whom died early in life. She was heartbroken by the death of her children and decided to honor their memory by devoting her life to improving the health of children and their mothers. She left her husband and began her nursing work as a public health nurse in Boston and Washington, D.C. while awaiting a post with the American Red Cross in France.

While in France, she worked tirelessly to provide food and healthcare to children, nursing mothers, and pregnant women. During this time, she became convinced that such a program could improve the health of mothers and children in rural America. She saw the advantages provided by trained midwives in Europe and thought the same preparation should be possible for nurses in the United States. She prepared herself by studying as a public health nurse at Teachers College, Columbia University, and then she studied midwifery, the profession or practice of assisting women during childbirth, at three British institutions.

Mary was deeply religious and considered this path to care for mothers and children to be her life's calling. In 1925, having been prepared as a nurse midwife and having studied the delivery of care in rural areas in Europe, she returned to the U.S. to try out her plan in rural Kentucky. She believed that she could improve the care provided in these underserved rural communities by preparing nurse midwives. She founded the Frontier Nurse Service with 2 colleagues she recruited from the United Kingdom.

The nurse midwives traveled by horseback to deliver babies and tend to their mothers day and night, in all weather. She obtained funding for the Frontier Nursing Service from wealthy friends of her family. Mary built her dream around a large log house, called "The Big House", in Wendover, Kentucky, and the nurses on horseback served the community from several clinic outposts. Within five years of opening the Frontier Nursing Service, the nurses had reached more than 1,000 families.

Nurse Breckinridge's legacy remains strong. "The Big House" in Wendover remains a central gathering place for students of the Frontier Nursing University, a school that now prepares more nurse midwives that any other nurse midwifery program in the United States. She was the pioneer who developed nurse midwifery in the United States and will always be known as the driving force behind rural health care in America.

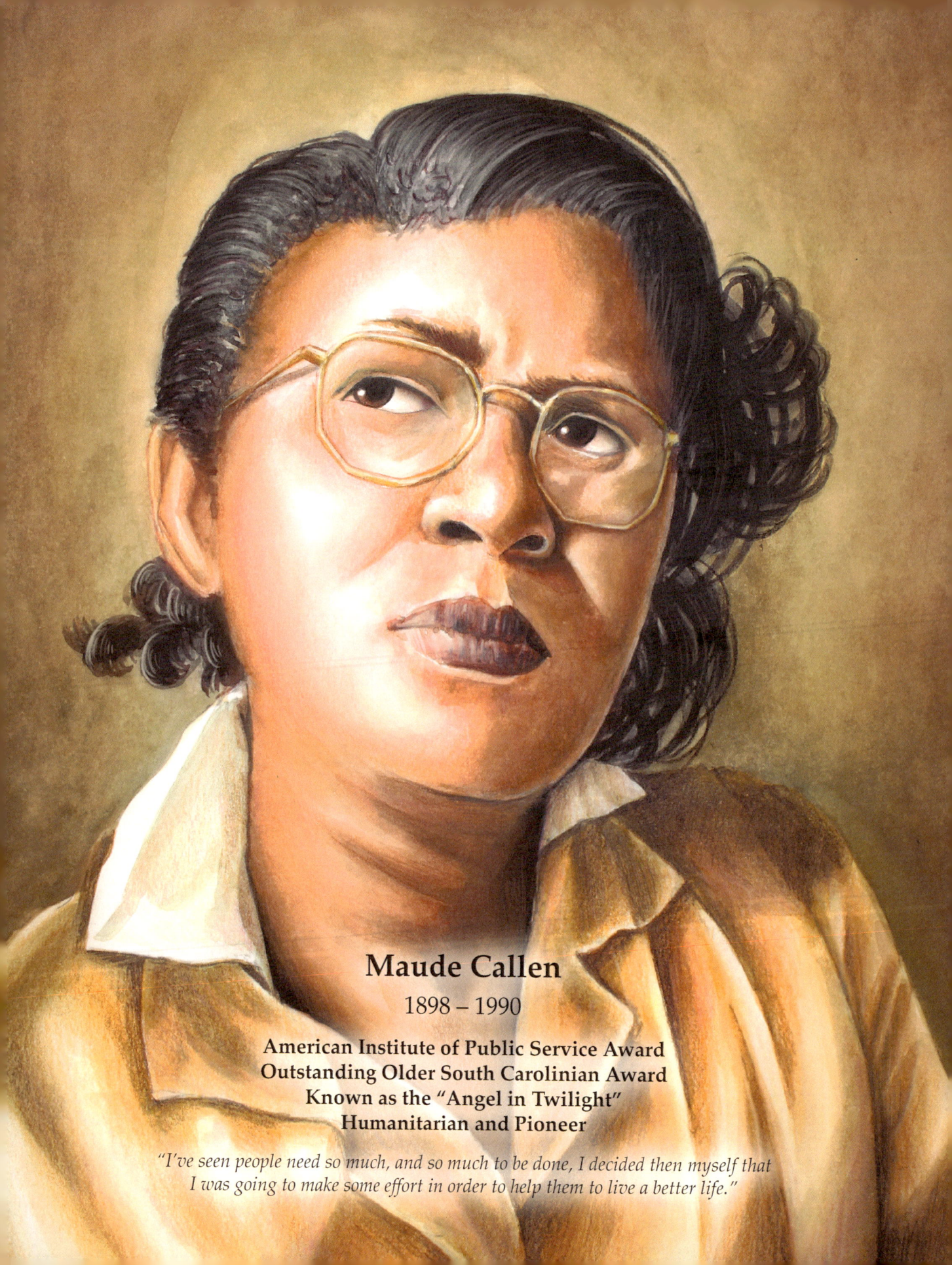

Maude Callen

1898 – 1990

**American Institute of Public Service Award
Outstanding Older South Carolinian Award
Known as the "Angel in Twilight"
Humanitarian and Pioneer**

*"I've seen people need so much, and so much to be done, I decided then myself that
I was going to make some effort in order to help them to live a better life."*

Maude Callen was born in 1898 in Tallahassee, Florida. She had twelve sisters and was orphaned at the age of 6. She then went to live with her uncle, who was the first black doctor in Tallahassee. He was inspirational to her as she decided to pursue a career in nursing. Maude went to Florida A&M and Tuskegee Institute and graduated with her nursing degree. She received additional training from the Georgia Infirmary in Savannah and in tuberculosis care at the Homer G. Phillips Hospital in St. Louis, Missouri.

After graduating, she went to Pineville, South Carolina, as a missionary nurse. In the early 1900s, healthcare was nonexistent in many poor and rural communities. People who lived farther away from major cities did not have hospitals or access to healthcare. Medical missions would set up makeshift tents or clinics to help the people living in the area. As part of the mission in Pineville, South Carolina, Nurse Callen provided nursing and midwifery care to thousands. She saw that there was so much to do in this area of the world due to its limited resources. She was driven to improve conditions and help the many people of rural South Carolina. By 1923, she had set up her own practice as a nurse midwife in Berkeley County, one of the poorest counties in South Carolina.

Nurse Callen was known to many as the "angel in twilight" because when she went to visit her patients in backwoods areas, she would have to bring her own lantern. Some of her patients did not have electricity or any light source. She would be seen walking over mud, fallen logs, and possibly dangerous areas, carrying her lantern so she could effectively examine her patients and provide the care that was needed. Maude also believed in educating people in her community to be nurses and midwives, so she passed her knowledge and training on to others.

In 1951, *Life Magazine* published a twelve-page essay about Maude Callen and her selfless work as a nurse midwife in rural South Carolina. The photo essay showed Maude working and highlighted her important work. This exposure helped Nurse Callen receive thousands of dollars in donations. She was then able to establish a modern clinic, the first of its kind in rural South Carolina. Maude worked at this clinic up until 1971, but she never stopped working to help those in her community. As a nurse midwife, during her more than 62 years of service as a midwife, she delivered over 600 babies.

After her retirement in 1971, Nurse Callen petitioned county officials to start a Senior Citizens Nutrition Site, which operated, starting in 1980, out of the clinic. As a volunteer, Maude managed the center, which cooked and delivered meals 5 days a week. She also provided car service to seniors needing transportation. At 85 years of age, she was still delivering meals to more than 50 other elderly residents, many of them younger than herself. She is said to have turned down an invitation from President Ronald Reagan to visit the White House, saying she had to do her job.

She continued her volunteer work until her death in 1990. She received recognition for her many volunteer works, including two honorary doctorates and several civic citations. Maude's perseverance to establish public health, educate the community, and give to those less fortunate is a long-lasting legacy. Nurse Maude Callen will be known as an "angel in twilight" for centuries to come.

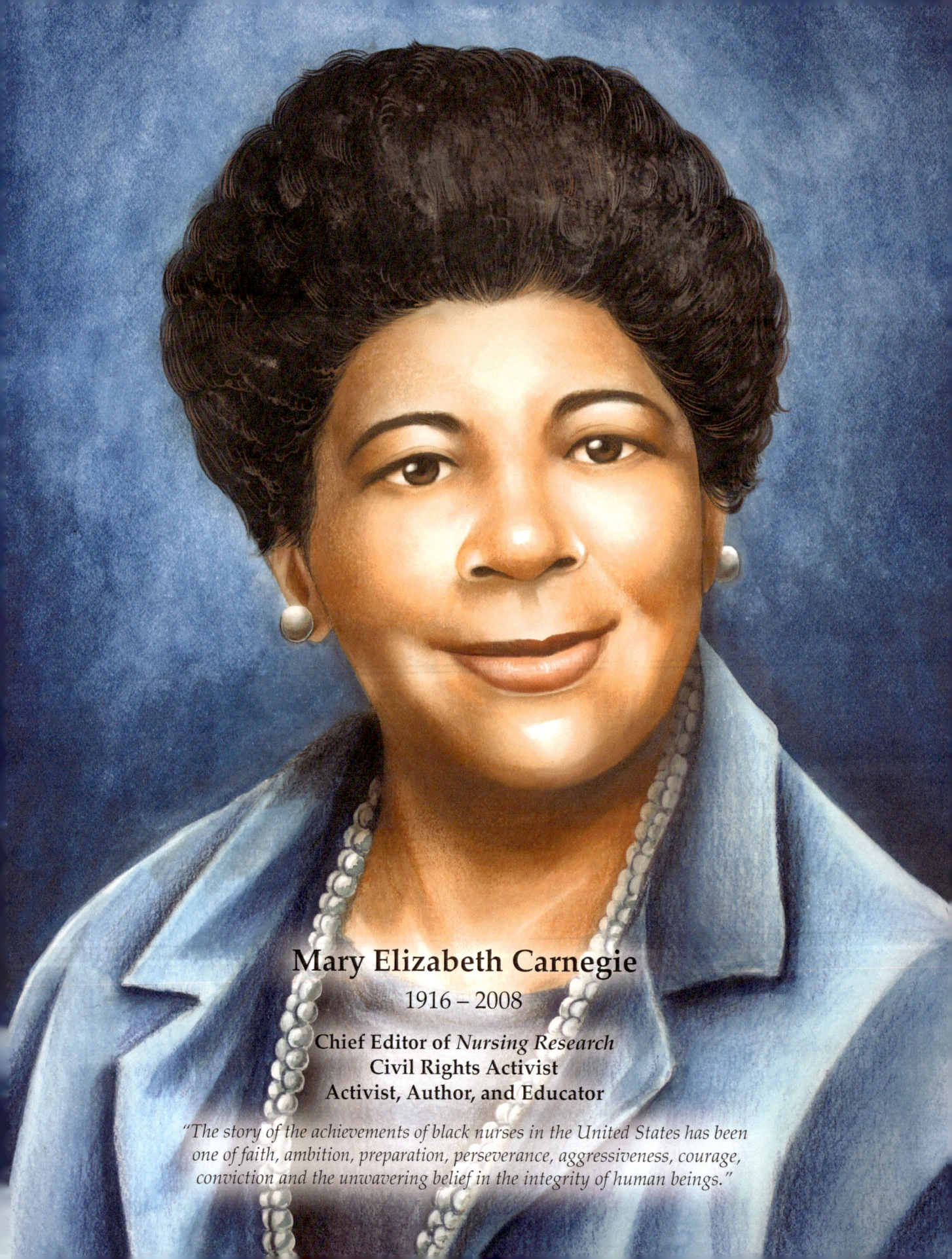

Mary Elizabeth Carnegie

1916 – 2008

Chief Editor of *Nursing Research*
Civil Rights Activist
Activist, Author, and Educator

"The story of the achievements of black nurses in the United States has been one of faith, ambition, preparation, perseverance, aggressiveness, courage, conviction and the unwavering belief in the integrity of human beings."

Mary Elizabeth Lancaster Carnegie was born to musician John Oliver and Adeline Swan Lancaster in Baltimore, Maryland, on April 19, 1916. Her parents divorced when she was 2 years old. She moved in with her maternal aunt and uncle and lived in Washington, D.C. Her aunt encouraged Mary's reading at an early age, and she entered kindergarten at the age of 4. She grew up happy, unaware of the segregation in the United States. This became obvious to her when she worked at a white cafeteria during high school and was unable to eat there herself.

Mary moved to New York City and enrolled in the Lincoln Hospital School of Nursing. She graduated in 1937. She began her clinical nursing career in the Veterans Hospital in Tuskegee, Alabama, and then practiced in several other hospitals. West Virginia State College offered to cover the cost of her education to obtain an undergraduate degree in return for her serving as a school nurse, so she pursued this education.

Mary never stopped learning and continued her education at several universities. She knew that she would need the academic credentials to combat the discrimination she would encounter in her career.

She received a Certificate in Administration in Schools of Nursing from the University of Toronto, a Master of Administration in Higher Education from Syracuse University, and a Doctor of Public Administration degree from New York University. While a student in Toronto, Mary met and married Eric Carnegie. They had a long-distance marriage for 10 years, which ended in divorce after they decided that neither one wanted to move to the other's city.

Mary taught nursing school after graduating from West Virginia State College at St. Phillip Hospital School of Nursing in Richmond, Virginia. It was two schools but was run by one administration, and the opportunities to learn how to take care of patients were different for black students. The hospitals were segregated in the south, as were the schools in the 1940s. The black hospitals could be a far distance from the black nursing schools. This was because of the "Jim Crow Laws" that determined where black citizens could eat, rest, live, learn, and receive healthcare. Black students were called by their first names, and white students were referred to as "Miss" or "Mrs."

Nurse Carnegie created a path for many to follow. She served as the editor of the *American Journal of Nursing*, which is the oldest professional nursing journal. She served as chief editor of the prestigious journal *Nursing Research* and was the first African American President of the American Academy of Nursing. She held many leadership roles in academic institutions.

Nurse Mary Elizabeth Carnegie was a pathfinder, serving as a leader in many capacities within the nursing profession, often being the first African American nurse to serve in leadership roles in the highest ranks of the profession. She was a mentor to many nurse leaders throughout the country. She owned a large co-op apartment in New York City, near Carnegie Hall, that served as the meeting place for nurses from around the United States who came to New York for professional meetings. She hosted several brainstorming sessions with these nurse leaders, questioning how things were and carving new paths for others to follow.

She worked tirelessly to advance knowledge and recognition of black nurse leaders. She was the author of three editions of the book *The Path We Tread: Blacks in Nursing Worldwide, 1854-1994*. She has been acclaimed as the champion of African American nurses, and she was a tireless advocate and leader on their behalf. Clear a path she did!

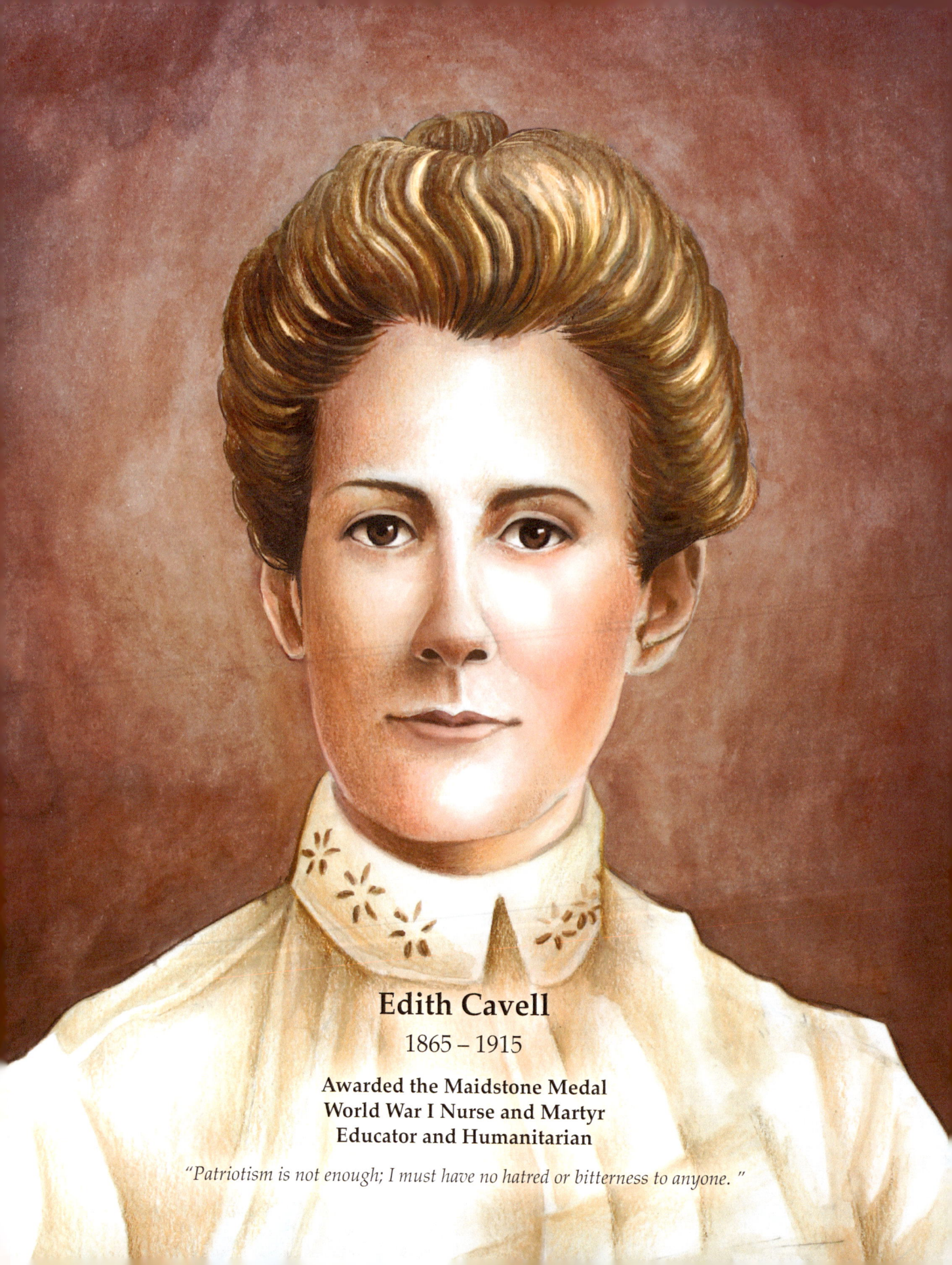

Edith Cavell

1865 – 1915

**Awarded the Maidstone Medal
World War I Nurse and Martyr
Educator and Humanitarian**

"Patriotism is not enough; I must have no hatred or bitterness to anyone."

Edith Louisa Cavell was born on December 4, 1865, in Swardeston, England, where her father was the pastor of the local church. Edith was the oldest of four children born to Louisa Sophia Warming and Reverend Frederick Cavell. Edith had a loving and gentle nature and felt a great sense of duty at an early age. She loved to paint flowers and speak French, and she was an outstanding student. Edith's proficiency in French proved helpful when she moved to Belgium to become a governess to the Francois family.

While working in Belgium, Edith's father became extremely ill, so she returned home to England to care for him. The experience of nursing her father back to health inspired Edith to pursue nursing. She began her professional training at Royal London Hospital in 1896. Edith was one of the nurses sent to Maidstone, a village about 30 miles east of London, because a typhoid epidemic had broken out. Typhoid is a bacterial infection that is passed through contaminated food and drinking water and is very contagious. Due to the poor sanitary conditions of the time, 1,847 people became infected, and 232 villagers died. The nurses were credited with saving many lives due to their attention to hand washing, food preparation, and other sanitation practices. Edith was one of many awarded the "Maidstone Medal," which was given by the townspeople in gratitude for the nurses' service.

Nurse Cavell held many positions in England and was well known for her organizational skills, teaching ability, and excellent bedside care. Dr. Antoine Depage, a Belgian surgeon, recruited Edith to head the nursing school he wanted to establish in Belgium. He was concerned that the Belgian nurses were not receiving the most current information, which was based on the work of Florence Nightingale. Edith had to be diplomatic, as she was an English Protestant woman assuming the responsibility for running the nursing schools from the Roman Catholic sisters who had been in charge for years. The school, named L'Ecole Belge d'Infirmieres Diplomees, was a great success.

When World War I began, Edith began working in a Red Cross Hospital, and she instructed the nurses to care for all of the soldiers without judgement, regardless of nationality. When the Germans invaded Belgium, the British and French troops were driven out, leaving many stranded soldiers behind. Nurse Cavell hid two British soldiers for two weeks at the nursing school and then helped them escape to Holland. Soon, other soldiers were seeking her help. Edith had a moral decision to make. As a "protected" member of the Red Cross, she needed to remain uninvolved, but she believed that she had an obligation, as a nurse, to save the soldiers by helping them escape. She worked with a network of people who assisted in providing safe passage to many soldiers. The Germans became suspicious of Edith, and a Belgian spy reported her to the German authorities. She was arrested on August 5, 1915. Despite the public outrage to free her, Edith was found guilty of treason and was sentenced to death. Edith died by a firing squad on October 12, 1915.

Nurse Cavell's execution prompted the Allied soldiers to fight even harder to honor her memory. Once the war was over, Edith's body was returned to England for a proper memorial service, which thousands of people attended. Edith's sense of duty from a young age allowed her to have no regrets about helping the desperate soldiers. A mountain is named after her and is located in Jasper National Park in Alberta, Canada, and a statue of her likeness is near Trafalgar Square in London.

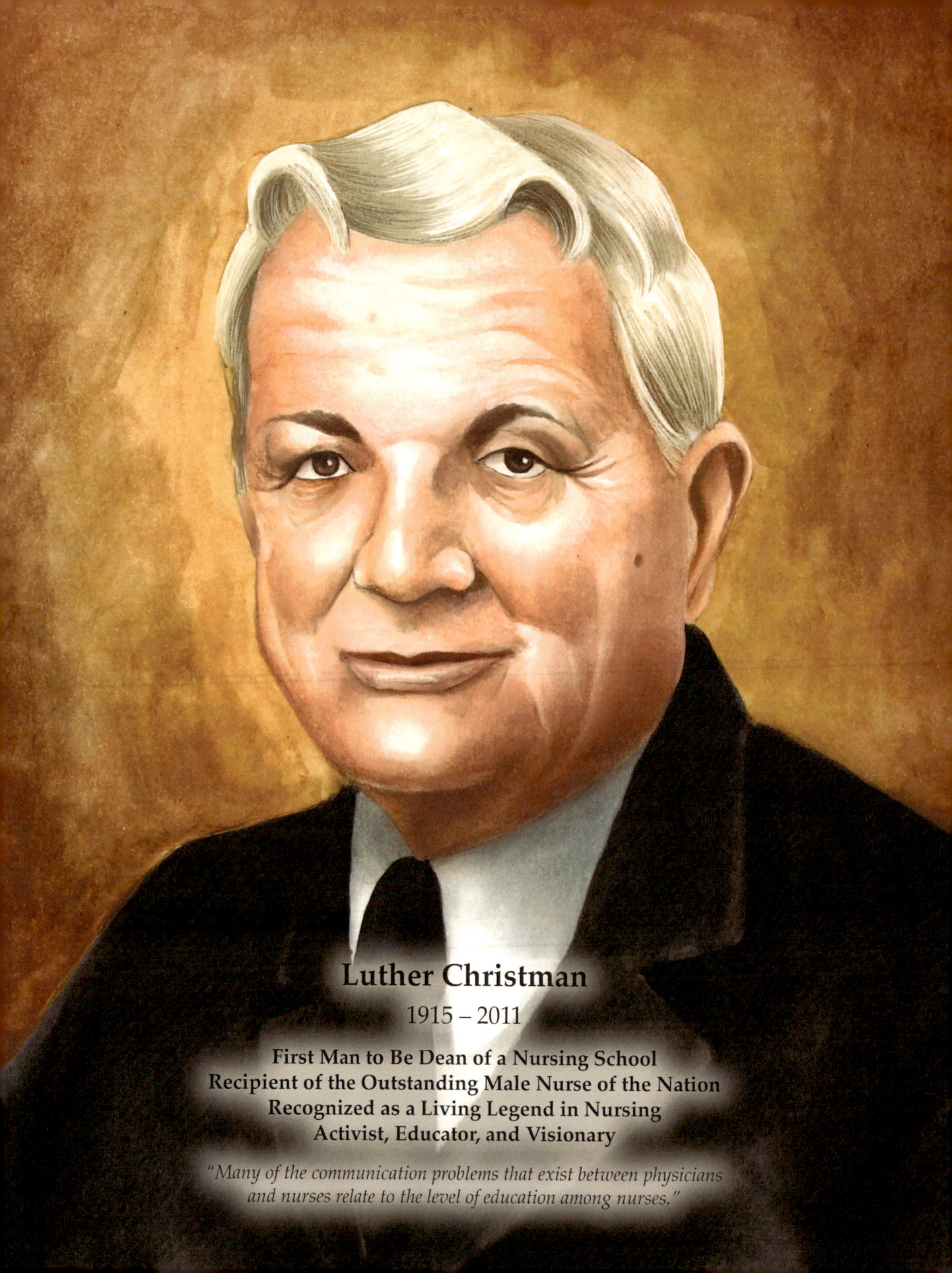

Luther Christman

1915 – 2011

**First Man to Be Dean of a Nursing School
Recipient of the Outstanding Male Nurse of the Nation
Recognized as a Living Legend in Nursing
Activist, Educator, and Visionary**

*"Many of the communication problems that exist between physicians
and nurses relate to the level of education among nurses."*

Luther Christman was born in Summit Hill, Pennsylvania, a farming and coal mining town, on February 26, 1915, and he was the first child in his family to survive infancy. Luther had a difficult childhood; his mother physically abused him and enrolled him in school at the age of 4 so that he could graduate early and help support the family. His father was a gentle man but was controlled by his harsh wife. His grandmother was very affectionate and encouraged Luther in his studies. As the youngest student in his class, Luther struggled in school. He worked hard and became an excellent student.

Luther met his future wife, Dorothy, in 1932, when they were 17 years old. They were trying to decide what to do with their lives, as career choices were limited due to the Great Depression, a time when over 25 percent of people had no work. A Lutheran minister encouraged Luther to consider becoming a nurse.

Luther convinced Dorothy to become a nurse, too, and they attended different nursing schools. They worked as nursing assistants 12 hours a day for 6 days a week, receiving $10-12 a month in living expenses from the hospitals. Luther spent the first two years of his training in a hospital specializing in care of men with mental illnesses. The thinking at the time was that men were more suited to care for these patients, as their illnesses could cause them to become combative. Christman graduated from the Pennsylvania Hospital School of Nursing for Men in 1939. He did not work as a nurse immediately after graduation; instead, he worked as a postal clerk because he could earn twice as much money.

He applied to several nursing colleges to continue his studies. Despite his impressive academic record, he was consistently rejected because of his gender. He felt defeated. In 1937, less than 1 percent of all nursing students were men. He was finally accepted to Temple University School of Nursing, although the discrimination continued. Because he was a man, he could not participate in maternity clinical rotations, and he was prevented from serving as an Army nurse during World War II despite there being a shortage of 2,000 nurses. After being nominated to run for president of the American Nurses Association and being favored to win, Luther was the victim of rumors that influenced the election. This prompted him to create a new professional organization now known as American Assembly for Men in Nursing in 1980.

Nurse Christman received a master's degree in clinical psychology in 1962, then a doctoral degree in anthropology and sociology. Luther believed that nursing should establish national educational standards for entry into practice and that nurses needed a solid education in the sciences and humanities to provide the highest quality of care.

Nurse Christman worked tirelessly to address diversity and gender inequality in nursing. He advocated for expanding the nursing role in patient care delivery. He was the first male dean of a major college of nursing when he became dean at Vanderbilt University in Nashville, Tennessee, in 1967. He implemented a unification model where professors of nursing and medicine taught nursing and medical students in the same classroom. He introduced the teacher-practitioner role, recognizing that the best teachers were those with advanced education who were caring for patients at the bedside. He left Vanderbilt and became dean of Rush University School of Nursing, where he led many reforms in nursing education and practice.

Luther Christman was a trailblazer; he left his unique handprint on many facets of nursing. Throughout his 65-year career in nursing, he challenged the current thinking of the time. He is one of nursing's most honored and celebrated leaders.

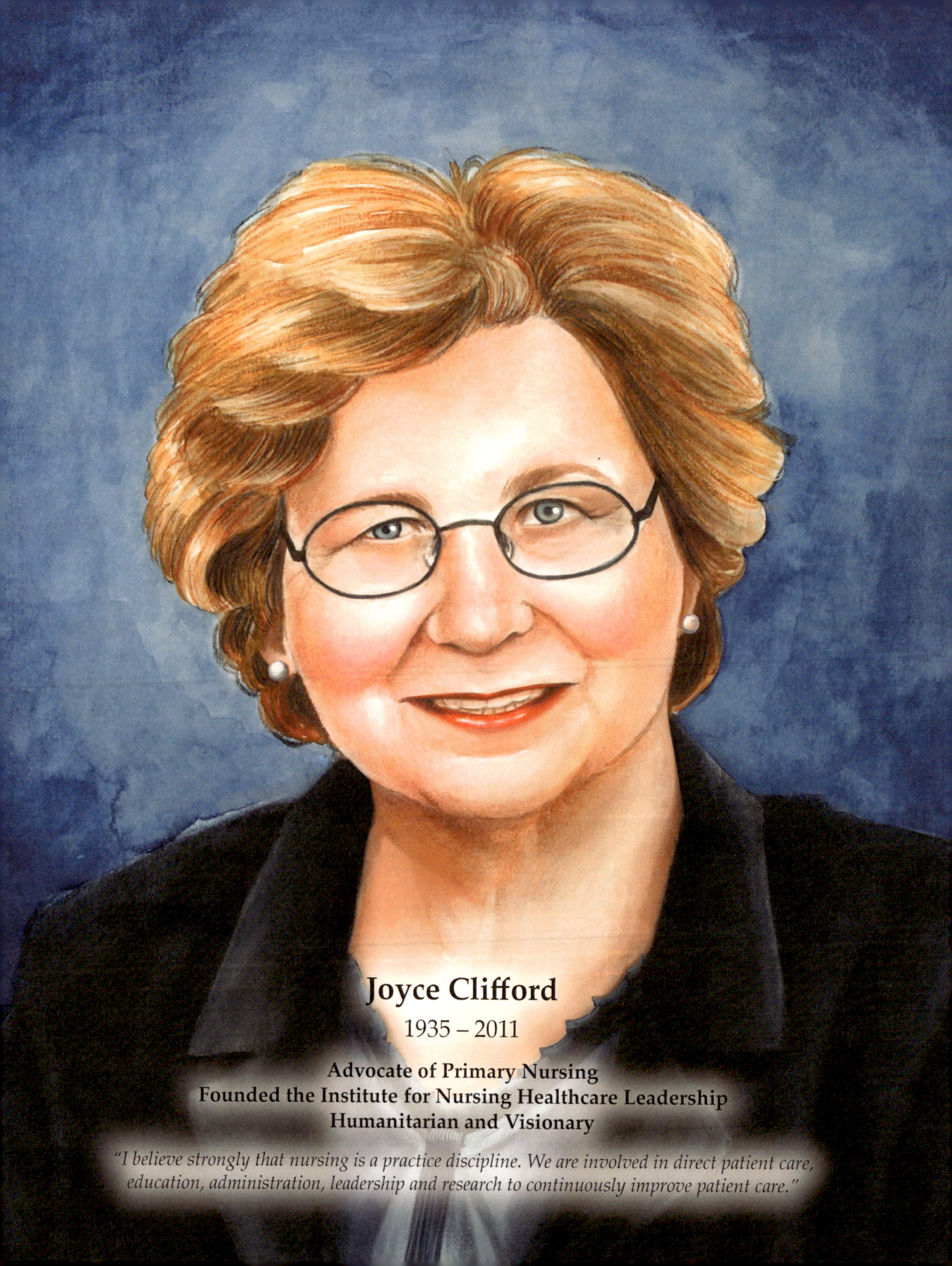

Joyce Clifford

1935 – 2011

Advocate of Primary Nursing
Founded the Institute for Nursing Healthcare Leadership
Humanitarian and Visionary

"I believe strongly that nursing is a practice discipline. We are involved in direct patient care,
education, administration, leadership and research to continuously improve patient care."

Joyce Hoyt Clifford is recognized as an exceptional nurse executive who created a hospital culture where nurses were respected, celebrated, and recognized for their expertise. Joyce was born on September 23, 1935, in New Haven, Connecticut. Joyce was the third of four girls born to Helen and Raymond Hoyt. Joyce's father, an iron worker, only completed the 10th grade, but he promoted the value of education to all of his daughters. Joyce was known for her fiery red hair, fear of public speaking, and mischievous nature. On her 16th birthday, Joyce obtained her Social Security card and work permit so that she could be hired as a nurse's aide at St. Raphael's Hospital. Joyce quickly discovered that taking care of people filled her heart with joy. Joyce so loved the opportunity to take care of others, that for just 35 cents an hour, she spent a Christmas Eve away from her family to take care of a young woman who was dying.

Joyce graduated from St. Raphael School of Nursing in New Haven and earned a Bachelor of Science in Nursing in nursing from St. Anselm College in New Hampshire in 1959. She returned to St. Raphael's as an instructor, where her fear of public speaking was put to the test. In her first anatomy and physiology lecture, she was so nervous that it took her only 45 minutes to present a lecture that should have taken 3 hours! She learned to conquer her fear and spoke to thousands of people all over the world during her 50-year career in nursing.

Joyce joined the Air Force Nurse Corps in the early 1960s and was stationed at Maxwell Air Force Base in Birmingham, Alabama, during the height of the Vietnam War. The Air Force provided Joyce with many lessons about leadership. She learned to appreciate the difference in rank but to make everyone feel equal, welcome different points of view, and invest time in the development of others. She met her husband, Lawrence Clifford, while attending the Master's in Nursing program at the University of Alabama. She earned the rank of major before leaving the Air Force.

Nurse Clifford held several different leadership positions at the University of Alabama and Indiana University before being recruited to Boston, Massachusetts. Serving as Senior Vice President and Nurse-in-Chief at Beth Israel Hospital, Joyce earned her reputation as a dynamic, innovative, and visionary leader. She implemented the role of the primary nurse, where the patient was assigned one nurse who was responsible for the nursing care during the patient's entire stay in the hospital. Joyce advocated for a partnership of equals between nurses and doctors. The nurses were recognized for their intellect, skill, and compassion. When Nurse Clifford arrived at Beth Israel, nurses would leave the hospital after working only three months. After several years of Joyce's leadership, qualified nurses were turned away because there were no openings.

While leading nursing practice at Beth Israel, Joyce earned a doctorate from Brandeis University in 1997. She left Beth Israel Hospital in 1999 and founded The Institute of Nursing Healthcare Leadership.

Nurse Clifford believed that leadership was not a title or position but how a person behaved. Joyce dedicated her career to influencing, respecting, and guiding nurses. As a result, her greatest legacy is the thousands of nurses she inspired to become leaders at the bedside as primary nurses and the hundreds she influenced to become mentors for the next generation of nurses.

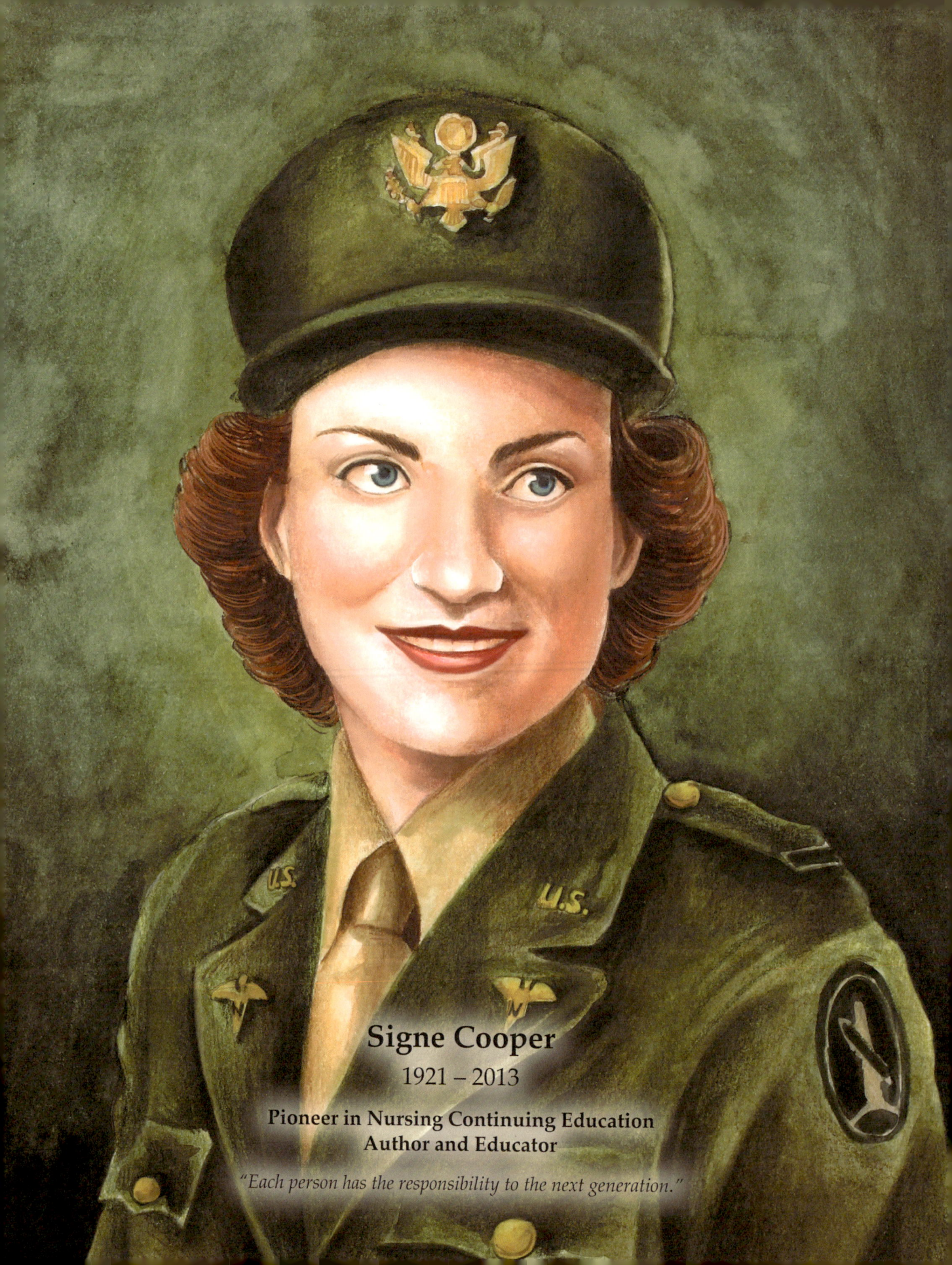

Signe Cooper

1921 – 2013

**Pioneer in Nursing Continuing Education
Author and Educator**

"Each person has the responsibility to the next generation."

Signe Skott was born in 1921 in Clinton County, Iowa. She was the second of four children born to Hans and Clara Steen Skott. She attended a one-room country school in Iowa through 8th grade. When Signe was 16, she and her family moved to Madison, Wisconsin. Signe's parents were farmers and were college-educated, which was something that was rare at the time. Signe's mother was the first woman in the town to drive a car. Her parents would engage Signe and her siblings by posing challenging questions in the evenings to see which child could come up with the right answer.

During the Great Depression, Signe's father became ill. He needed surgery, but the surgeon would not perform the surgery until her father had paid the bill in advance. Signe's family struggled to find the money for the surgery, until her mother persuaded Signe's uncle to provide the surgeon with a hog for payment. Signe's father recovered, but the ordeal left a lasting impression on Signe. She would never forget the doctor, his heartless bedside manner, and his refusal to help her father until he had been paid.

Signe completed high school and entered the University of Wisconsin-Madison to study nursing. While she was in college, World War II began, and the demand for nurses increased. In 1943, Signe volunteered for the Army Nurse Corps. She was first stationed in Virginia, where she received her military training, and then she was sent to India. It was her first plane ride, and it took her halfway across the world.

In India, she served as a 1st lieutenant in military hospitals in Leo and Margherita, India. She worked with patients who had been wounded, suffered from polio, or suffered from mental health disorders. It was intense work, and usually little could be done to save patients who had contagious diseases. The polio vaccine had not been created yet, and the antibiotic Penicillin had just become available. The nurses were not permitted to mix the antibiotic powder with the sterile water. That was a task the doctors needed to do. She remained in India until 1945. Signe married Clois Cooper, but the marriage ended in divorce.

Nurse Cooper returned to Wisconsin when her service as an Army nurse was complete. There, she took a job as a head nurse on an obstetrics unit. There were so many babies being born that the nurses often ran out of bassinets and had to place the newborns in baby bathtubs. She completed her nursing degree at the University of Wisconsin-Madison in 1948. Her clinical skills and knowledge were impressive, and Signe was asked to be an instructor at the nursing school.

Nurse Cooper earned a master's degree in education from the University of Wisconsin-Madison while continuing to teach. She introduced classes on death and dying and care of the elderly that had not been included as part of a nurse's education. In 1966, she delivered one of the first extension courses at the university, broadcasting lectures by telephone to over 600 students at 24 "listening post" locations across Wisconsin.

After her retirement, Signe developed a new field of expertise: nursing history. She collected the stories of hundreds of Wisconsin nurses and documented the history of the University of Wisconsin-Madison nursing school.

Nurse Signe Cooper believed in the power of learning and dedicated her career to creating novel educational programs and sharing her knowledge in publications. She earned several distinguished awards because of her commitment to the nursing profession. She donated her estate to the University of Wisconsin-Madison School of Nursing.

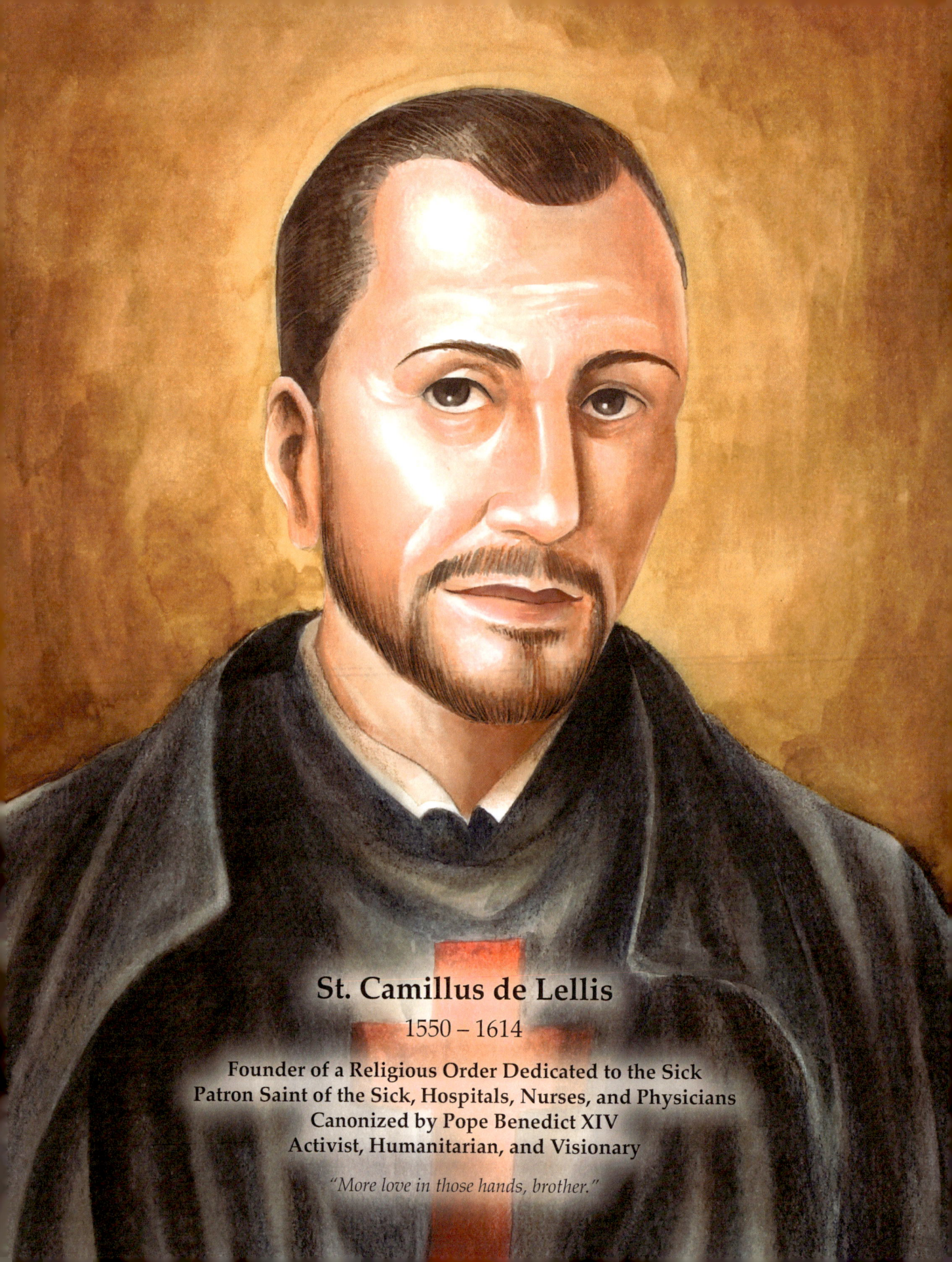

St. Camillus de Lellis

1550 – 1614

Founder of a Religious Order Dedicated to the Sick
Patron Saint of the Sick, Hospitals, Nurses, and Physicians
Canonized by Pope Benedict XIV
Activist, Humanitarian, and Visionary

"More love in those hands, brother."

Camillus de Lellis was born into a noble family on May 25, 1550, in Bucchianico, Italy. His mother died when he was 12 years old. Camillus disliked school and dropped out. He was 6 feet 6 inches by the age of 16, and having nothing to occupy his time, he joined his father in the Venetian army, fighting the Turks. He wounded his leg during a battle, which resulted in an injury that caused him pain and suffering the rest of his life. Like his father, Camillus had a terrible temper and a love of gambling. This habit would result in Camillus becoming penniless, losing everything he owned, including his boots.

Needing money, Camillus took a job as a workman at a Capuchin Monastery. Despite his aggressive nature and excessive gambling, the head Monk, or Guardian, of the monastery tried to nurture the kind and gentle side of Camillus that he had noticed in him. Deciding to change his life for the better, Camillus hoped to become a monk, but his diseased leg and lack of education prevented him from doing so. Three times he attempted to join the monastery, and three times he was turned away.

Seeking medical attention for his leg, Camillus entered St. Giacomo Hospital in Rome. In the mid-1500s, there was little in the way of medicines or treatments that could help heal Camillus's leg ulcer, and his condition was declared incurable by his doctors. To pay for his hospital stay, he began to care for other patients. Suffering himself, Camillus was distraught by what he saw and decided to improve the care and surroundings for his patients.

The nurses caring for the patients in the hospital were all men. They were insensitive to their patients' suffering, often disrespectful, and left the men uncleaned. The hospital was dirty, and there was an offensive odor that lingered in the patient rooms and hallways. Because of poor ventilation and no handwashing between patients, diseases spread easily. Camillus went on to become the director of the St. Giacomo Hospital but was unable to implement the changes he had dreamed of making.

Camillus believed that he was called to create a religious order that would be dedicated to caring exclusively for the sick. He began to study at the Jesuit Roman College and was ordained as a priest in 1584. He created The Ministers of the Sick, more popularly known as "The Camillians," with two companions. They wore black cassocks and ankle-length robes, and a large red cross was sewn on the front of their robes, positioned over their hearts. This was to distinguish them from soldiers on the battlefield. They are credited with creating the first field medical unit.

His order expanded, and there were many men seeking religious lives who also felt called to care for the sick. They began their work at the hospital of Santo Spiritu in Rome. Father de Lellis insisted that the members of his order be well educated in the care of the sick. He demanded that each patient be treated with compassion, respect, and thoughtfulness. He was attentive to the hospital environment, isolating patients who were contagious. He required that food being offered to patients was nutritious and would aid in their recovery. Father de Lellis took care of the sickest patients and would crawl to visit his patients when he was unable to walk.

Father de Lellis raised the standard of care for those needing medical attention. Today, the Camillians serve in over 91 hospitals in 42 countries. They own and operate health centers, universities, and education centers.

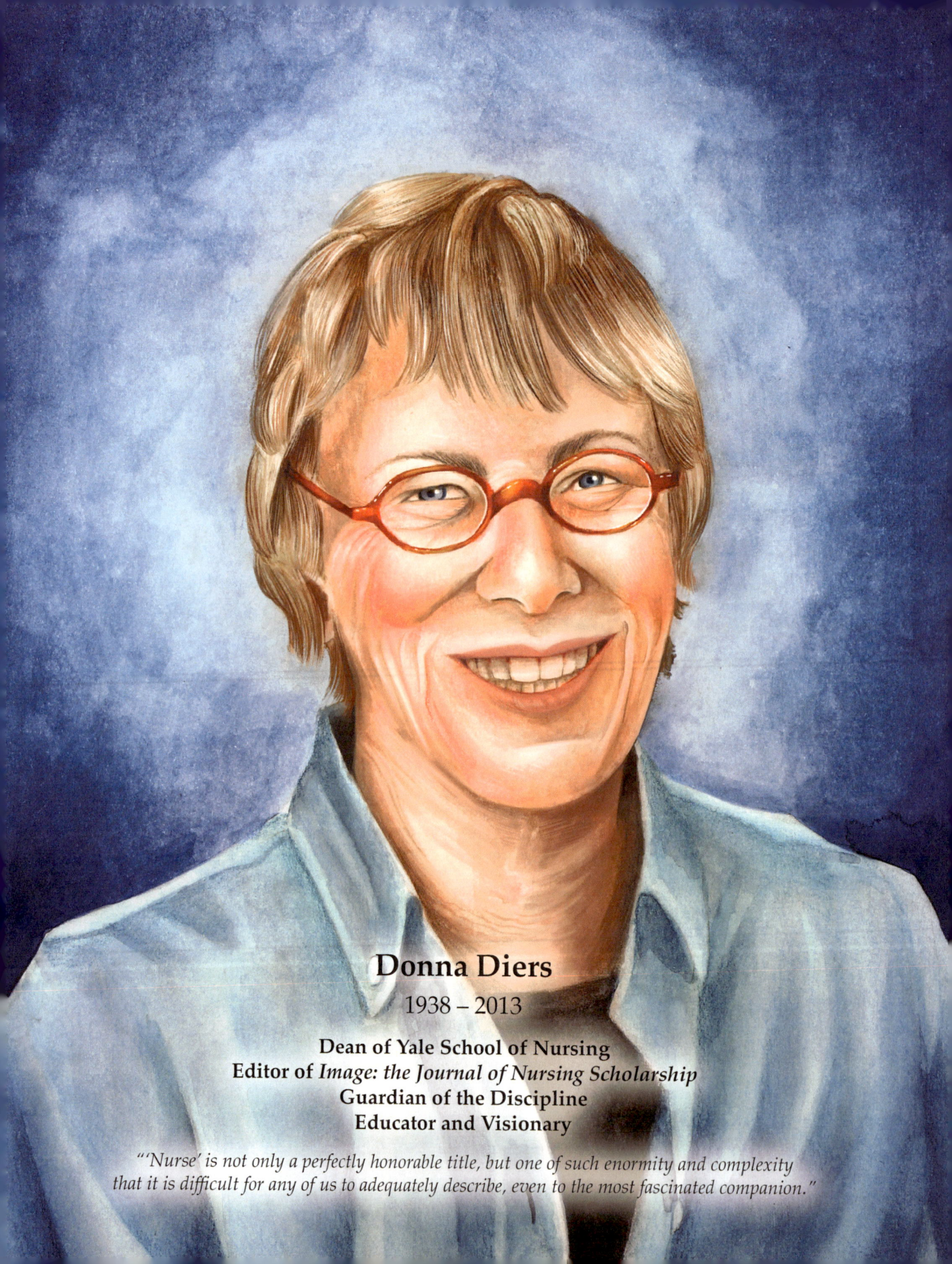

Donna Diers

1938 – 2013

Dean of Yale School of Nursing
Editor of *Image: the Journal of Nursing Scholarship*
Guardian of the Discipline
Educator and Visionary

*"'Nurse' is not only a perfectly honorable title, but one of such enormity and complexity
that it is difficult for any of us to adequately describe, even to the most fascinated companion."*

Donna Kaye Diers was born on May 11, 1938, in Sheridan, Wyoming. Her mother and father, Ilene and Don, loved to read, and they passed the passion on to their 2 children. Donna and her younger brother, Jim, would spend their childhood summers riding their bikes to the local library. Donna checked out the maximum books allowed, which was 7, every week. She would read books to her brother and his friends in the backyard. Donna loved words and wanted to be a journalist. Her mother encouraged her to take a typing course if she really wanted to be a writer. She dropped out of the class before mastering the number line and always had to look down at the keyboard to locate the $, %, and @ keys.

Donna fell into nursing after watching the mother of one of her neighbor's friends, named Georgia, come home from work. Georgia would pull into the driveway after her shift, dressed in her spotless white uniform, polished white shoes, white stockings, and a nursing cap. In the summertime, before she would go into the house, Georgia would go into the backyard, take off her uniform, and hang it on the clothesline outside. She was caring for patients with polio. It was the 1950s, and polio was infecting and paralyzing thousands of children. Polio was one of the most feared contagious viral illnesses, and it caused nerve injury that lead to paralysis, difficulty breathing, and occasionally death. Donna knew the importance of Georgia's work because her best friend, Beth, had polio, and Georgia would also look after her.

Donna graduated from the University of Denver with her undergraduate nursing degree in 1960. She got her master's in nursing from Yale University and her PhD from the University of Technology in Sydney, Australia. She served as Dean of the Yale School of Nursing from 1972-1985. While Dean, Nurse Diers accomplished many things. She created the first graduate program in nursing that did not require an undergraduate degree in nursing. She led the development of advanced practice nursing. Advanced practice nurses hold master's or doctoral degrees in nursing and provide primary health and preventive care services to the public. She advocated for nurses to be thinkers, researchers, and scientists. She wrote one of the first textbooks about nursing research. She was the editor of *Image: the Journal of Nursing Scholarship* for 8 years.

Of all of her many accomplishments, her most remarkable contribution to the profession of nursing was her writing. She didn't become a journalist, because she was too timid, but her ability to use just the right word in just the right order in just the right sentence was poetic. It would have made any true journalist jealous. In an editorial titled "Excellence in Nursing," Donna wrote, *"Nurses deal with the most basic of human needs: feeding, heartbreak, warmth, elimination, suffering, loneliness, birth and death. Our hands get dirty, our uniforms stained and our psyches eroded by the daily contact with human beings in need – people crying, immobilized, angry, frightened, depressed and only occasionally joyful… With our hands and eyes, we touch the lives of others and are admitted to the privacy of their inner space without even asking."*

While Donna described herself as a very shy and private person, she found it within herself to be bold when it came to advocating for the profession of nursing. She encouraged nurses to become politically active and to get involved in policy-making decisions. Nurse Donna Diers made nursing visible through her writings, teachings, and mentoring, and she taught future generations of nurses to do the same.

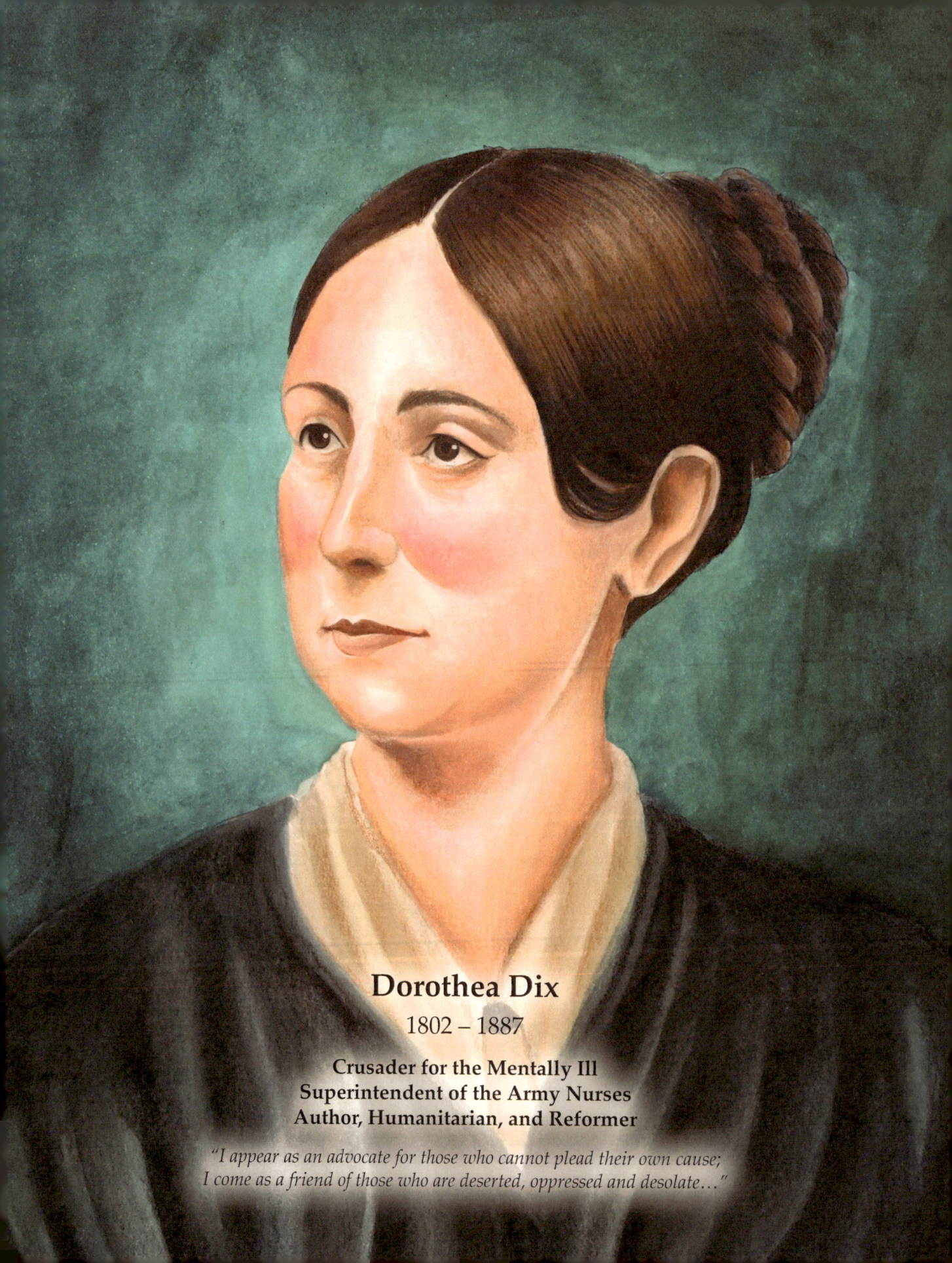

Dorothea Dix

1802 – 1887

Crusader for the Mentally Ill
Superintendent of the Army Nurses
Author, Humanitarian, and Reformer

"I appear as an advocate for those who cannot plead their own cause;
I come as a friend of those who are deserted, oppressed and desolate…"

Dorothea Lynde Dix was born on April 4, 1802, to Joseph and Mary Bigelow Dix. She grew up in the small village of Hampden, Maine, the oldest of three children. Dorothea grew up lonely and felt abandoned, as her mother experienced depression and was unable to care for her and her brothers. Dorothea's father had a temper and struggled with alcoholism. Her parents depended on her to take care of her younger siblings. At the age of 12, Dorothea left home to move in with her wealthy paternal grandmother in Boston. Her grandmother was strong willed like Dorothea. They often disagreed, yet she was able to convince her grandmother to allow her to use a portion of their home to open a school for girls. Dorothea was 14 at the time.

Teaching was the only career available to single women in the early 1800s, and Dorothea was an excellent teacher. She spent her time out of the classroom learning; she attended lectures and classes to educate herself and was most interested in the sciences. She also believed that education should include religious and ethical principles. Her reputation as an educator grew throughout Boston, and she was recruited to teach at the Boston Female Monitorial School, where they were using new techniques like blackboards, maps, and written lessons.

At age 22, Dorothea became an author, publishing her most famous book, *Conversations on Common Things*, in 1824. This was quite an accomplishment, as it was rare for a woman to be published. Dorothea wrote the book as if a mother and daughter were having a conversation and the mother was offering advice about living a fulfilling life, which was something she never experienced with her own mother.

Dorothea continued to educate girls, opening another school in 1831. She was a dedicated teacher and spent hours preparing lessons, so much so that she was not taking care of herself and became ill. Her friends encouraged her to take time off, and she went to England to rest. While she was there, she met two activists working to reform prisons and care for the mentally ill.

Upon her return to the United States, she decided to devote her life to charitable work. She was able to support herself because her grandmother had left her an inheritance. She began volunteering as a Sunday school teacher in a prison. During her visits, she saw people with mental illnesses chained to walls; they were cold, malnourished, and without adequate clothing. They were left in the dark, neglected. She was stunned and outraged by what she observed. While women did not have the right to vote or hold political office, Dorothea used her exceptional organizational skills and began educating politicians on the horrific conditions. She lobbied for change and moral treatment for the mentally ill and traveled across the United States visiting prisons, mental institutions, and hospitals. She advocated for improvements in lighting, ventilation, heating, nutrition, and security and demanded that the special facilities for the mentally ill be staffed with educated, skilled, and compassionate staff.

When the American Civil War started, Dorothea volunteered to work as a nurse, although she had never received formal education as a nurse. She was asked to serve as the Superintendent of the Army Nurses in 1861. She was the first woman to hold an executive position in the United States government.

After the Civil War, Dorothea resumed her work to improve the conditions for mentally ill patients. Her work to provide equal and humane care for the mentally ill was groundbreaking. Her advocacy for equal and empathic treatment lives on today.

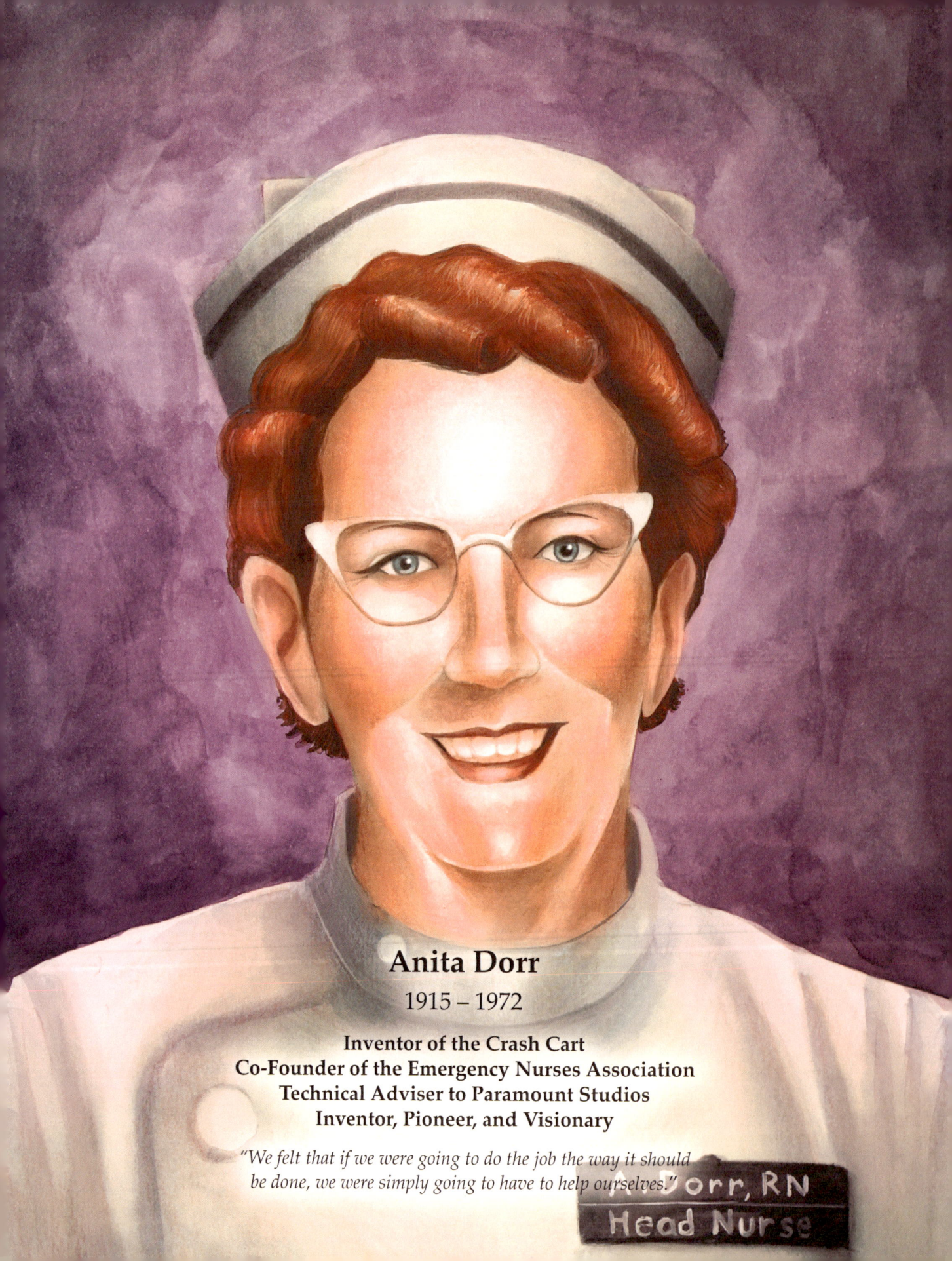

Anita Dorr

1915 – 1972

**Inventor of the Crash Cart
Co-Founder of the Emergency Nurses Association
Technical Adviser to Paramount Studios
Inventor, Pioneer, and Visionary**

*"We felt that if we were going to do the job the way it should
be done, we were simply going to have to help ourselves."*

A. Dorr, RN
Head Nurse

Anita Dowling Dorr was one of ten siblings; she was born on April 18, 1915, in Titusville, Pennsylvania. She had a fiery spirit, and even at a young age she was a force of nature. These traits served her well as she paved the way for emergency nurses to be recognized as a unique nursing specialty. Anita graduated from the Edward J. Meyer Memorial Hospital School of Nursing in Buffalo, New York. She began her career in the operating room and then joined the U.S. Army Nurse Corps at the age of 27 in 1942.

Her tours of duty took her to Africa and then to Europe, where she tended to wounded soldiers in Italy, France, and Germany during World War II. Anita was affected deeply by the experience of witnessing the liberation of the Jewish prisoners from the concentration camps and seeing the degree of suffering they had endured both physically and emotionally. She dedicated her career to providing nursing care that was holistic, compassionate, and equitable. She achieved the rank of captain before leaving the Army. Anita returned to Buffalo and married John Dorr. They had two children.

Anita brought her military training and leadership skills to the Emergency and Admissions Department when she assumed the Supervisor position at the Edward J. Meyer Memorial Hospital in 1960. She was decisive, efficient, and stern. It was said that she ran the departments with military precision. She insisted that she be called "Mrs. Dorr," and no one ever made the mistake of calling her Anita more than once.

The Emergency Room (ER) of the 1960s was nothing similar to what is shown on television and in the movies of today. CPR, the emergency life-saving procedure, was beginning to be used in 1960. Anita noticed that the ER nurses were spending precious time gathering equipment to take with them as they responded to emergencies or "codes" throughout the hospital. She and her husband designed the "crisis cart" in their garage, and it contained all of the essential equipment and medicines needed in a "code." The cart was painted red and was placed on wheels so that it could be moved easily and quickly. It also contained a bicycle bell to alert the staff to move out of the way. Anita never applied for a patent for the "crisis cart" because the legal advice she was given discouraged her from doing so. Unfortunately, Anita and her husband never benefited financially from their invention.

Emergency care was changing rapidly. Doctors and nurses who had served in World War II and in Vietnam were bringing their knowledge and experience to the ERs about what could be done on the battlefield to treat and stabilize patients before sending them to the hospital. Anita implemented a program in which ER nurses rode in ambulances to begin treatment at the accident scene, which increased the patient's chances of survival. Anita's superior knowledge of the ER was so well known that Paramount Studios hired her to serve as a technical adviser to ensure accurate portrayal of emergency situations in their media productions.

Anita realized that ER nurses needed additional knowledge and skills to deliver state of the science care to every patient who came through the ER doors. Just like every time she saw a problem, she fixed it. The Emergency Nurses' Association, which she co-created out of her garage with Judy Kelleher, an ER nurse from California, started with 3,400 members. It has grown to over 50,000 ER nurses today. Sadly, Anita died a week before the first national meeting was held in her hometown. ER nurses thrive today because of her amazing vision.

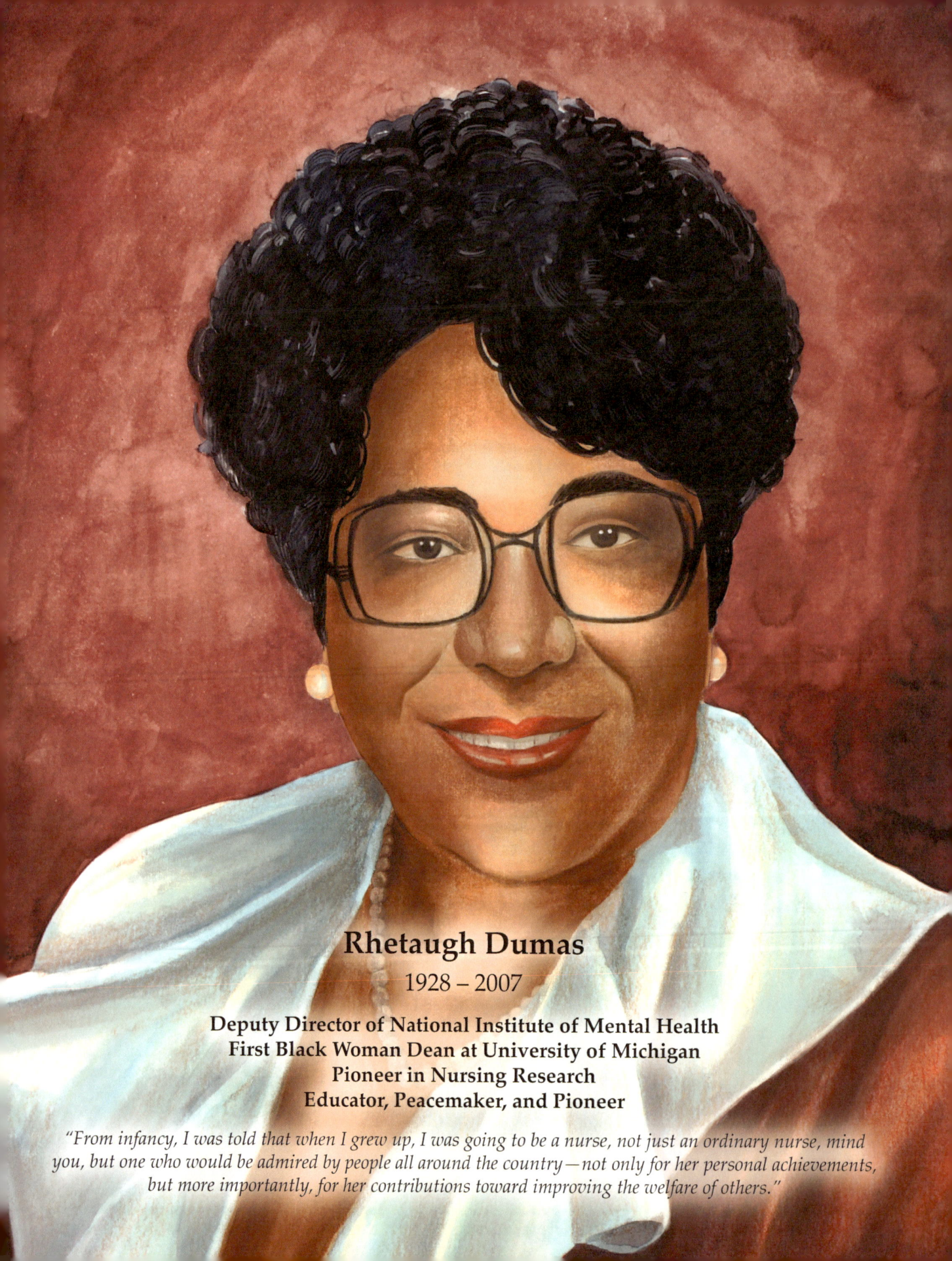

Rhetaugh Dumas

1928 – 2007

**Deputy Director of National Institute of Mental Health
First Black Woman Dean at University of Michigan
Pioneer in Nursing Research
Educator, Peacemaker, and Pioneer**

"From infancy, I was told that when I grew up, I was going to be a nurse, not just an ordinary nurse, mind you, but one who would be admired by people all around the country—not only for her personal achievements, but more importantly, for her contributions toward improving the welfare of others."

Rhetaugh Graves Dumas was born in 1928 in Natchez, Mississippi, to Josephine Clemmons and Rhetaugh Graves. Rhetaugh loved to sing and had a glorious voice, but nursing was her dream. She was inspired by her mother, who always wanted to be a nurse but was prevented because of the obstacles of the time. There were no nursing schools near her mother's childhood home that admitted African American women, and her grandparents did not have money to send her mother far from home.

Rhetaugh earned an undergraduate degree in nursing from Dillard University in New Orleans in 1951. Rhetaugh began her career as a substitute teacher in the segregated schools in Natchez and worked at Dillard University as the Director of the Student Health Center. She then traveled north and received a master's degree in psychiatric mental health nursing from Yale University. Rhetaugh married Albert Dumas, and they had one daughter, Adrienne Josephine. They were married for nine years.

Rhetaugh joined the nursing faculty at Yale University, and while teaching students, she conducted original research on how important nursing care is to patients who have just had surgery. She was the first nurse to use the scientific method, and her findings were important. She studied the effect of specific nursing actions that reduced stress and nausea in postoperative patients. This work is considered a "classic" within the nursing profession. While on the faculty at Yale, she also worked as Director of Nursing at the Connecticut Mental Health Center. She was a peacemaker during the school riots in the 1960s, helping mental health professionals provide counseling to parents and students in Hartford. Her concerns were particularly directed toward those who were from poor and underserved communities.

Beginning in the 1970s, Nurse Dumas was recruited to a leadership position at the National Institute of Mental Health (NIMH). While working at NIMH, Rhetaugh received a doctoral degree in social psychology from Union for Experimenting Colleges and Universities in 1975. She continued to use her knowledge and expertise of mental health to advance the needs of the underserved, overlooked, and vulnerable members of society. Her leadership was bold, focused, and inspiring, and as a result, Rhetaugh was the first nurse and African American woman to ever be promoted to the position of Deputy Director of the National Institute of Mental Health, a very important position in the United States government.

Following her work at NIMH, Nurse Dumas achieved another first when she was appointed as the first black woman to serve as Dean of Nursing at the University of Michigan. She also served in the Provost's office as Vice Provost for Health.

Nurse Dumas served as President of the American Academy of Nursing and the National League for Nursing. In 2002, she was named a Living Legend of the American Academy of Nursing, the highest honor bestowed by the prestigious organization.

Nurse Rhetaugh Dumas fulfilled her mother's prediction. She made the world better with her strength of convictions, her passion for the profession of nursing, and her dedication to those in need. One of her proudest accomplishments was being appointed by President Bill Clinton in 1996 to the National Bioethics Advisory Commission. In this role, she helped advise the president on bioethical issues arising from advances in science and technology. Rhetaugh had a majestic voice that commanded respect. While introducing herself to her colleagues on the Commission, whom she thought might have perceived her as a token appointee due to her gender, race, and professional background, she said, "I accepted President Clinton's invitation to join this Commission because I am eminently qualified to be here."

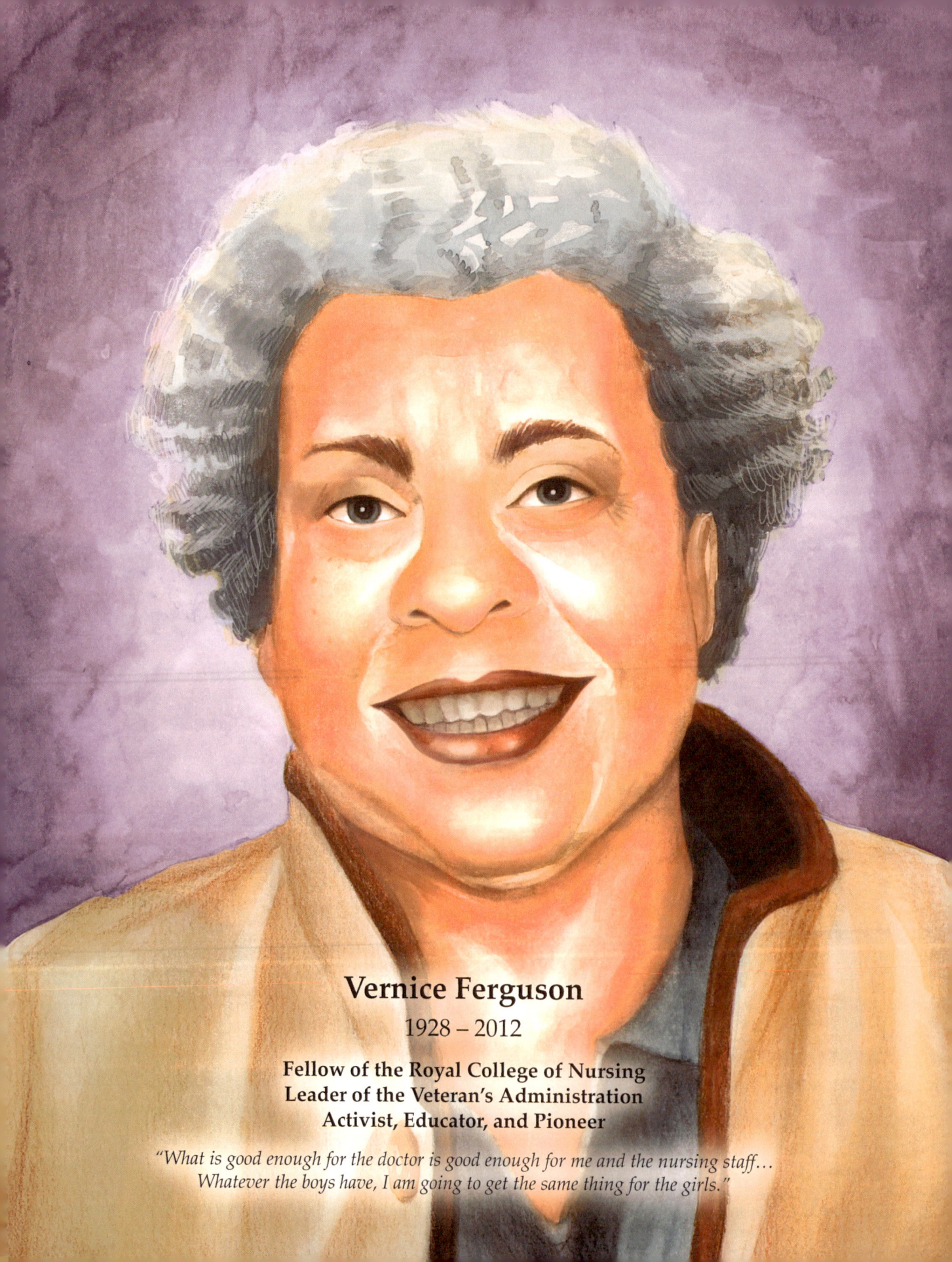

Vernice Ferguson

1928 – 2012

**Fellow of the Royal College of Nursing
Leader of the Veteran's Administration
Activist, Educator, and Pioneer**

*"What is good enough for the doctor is good enough for me and the nursing staff…
Whatever the boys have, I am going to get the same thing for the girls."*

Vernice Doris Ferguson was born June 13, 1928, in Fayetteville, North Carolina, the second of four children. Vernice grew up in Baltimore, Maryland, where her father was a minister and her mother was a teacher. Throughout her career, Vernice displayed talents she learned from both parents. She was a role model throughout her career, and she was a teacher at heart, challenging others to always do their best. Her speeches were memorable. She learned from her minister father how to deliver speeches filled with emotion and passion. Her voice commanded attention because of its strong, powerful, and authoritative quality, and her brilliant smile put people at ease. Vernice never missed an opportunity to inspire nurses and to promote the nursing profession to those who were not yet nurses.

As a child, Vernice grew up in a segregated city. Her home was open to friends and associates of her parents, and they stayed with her family because black individuals could not go to a hotel and spend the night. She recalled participating in exciting conversations at the dinner table, as the house guests would often share stories, raise important issues, and discuss their opinions about the latest books they had read.

Vernice's leadership skills were recognized early in life, first by her older sister, who accused Vernice of being "bossy," and later in middle school by her classmates, who always elected Vernice either president or treasurer because they knew that she would get things done. As a high school student, Vernice volunteered as a "candy striper." The outdated term described high school-aged girls who wore a pin-striped uniform and assisted staff with non-patient care duties in the hospital. This experience confirmed for Vernice that becoming a nurse was her ultimate career choice. Before becoming a nurse, Vernice taught high school science classes.

Vernice attended New York University, where she received her undergraduate nursing degree in 1950. At the graduation ceremony, when she was awarded the Lavinia Dock prize for high scholastic standing, the director of nursing refused to shake Vernice's extended hand. This disrespectful and insensitive act was witnessed by Vernice's family, who sat in the audience. Vernice later earned a master's degree from Teachers College, Columbia University.

Nurse Ferguson first worked as a nurse at the National Institutes of Health research unit at Montefiore Medical Center in the Bronx, New York. She then went on to work for several other hospitals. Her most important positions were both United States government related. She was the Chief Nurse at the National Institutes of Health Clinical Center from 1972 to 1980, and then she became the Chief Nurse at the Veteran's Administration (VA) from 1980 to 1992. In this position, she oversaw the largest nursing service in the world, with more than 60,000 nurses. She was recognized nationally for her leadership in this role, speaking up on behalf of nurses when the nation faced a national shortage of nurses. She spoke out about the critical and often unrecognized and underappreciated contribution of the nurse to patient care. She advocated for salary increases, demanding that the pay be equal to the life-saving responsibility of their positions.

Nurse Ferguson received many awards and led many professional nursing organizations and societies. She was the second American nurse to be named as an honorary Fellow of the Royal College of Nursing in the United Kingdom.

What distinguished Nurse Vernice Ferguson's contributions in the profession of nursing was her expectation of excellence. She was generous with her time while mentoring young nurses, tireless in her advocacy for advanced education and participation in nursing research, and enthusiastic about creating partnerships with other caregivers.

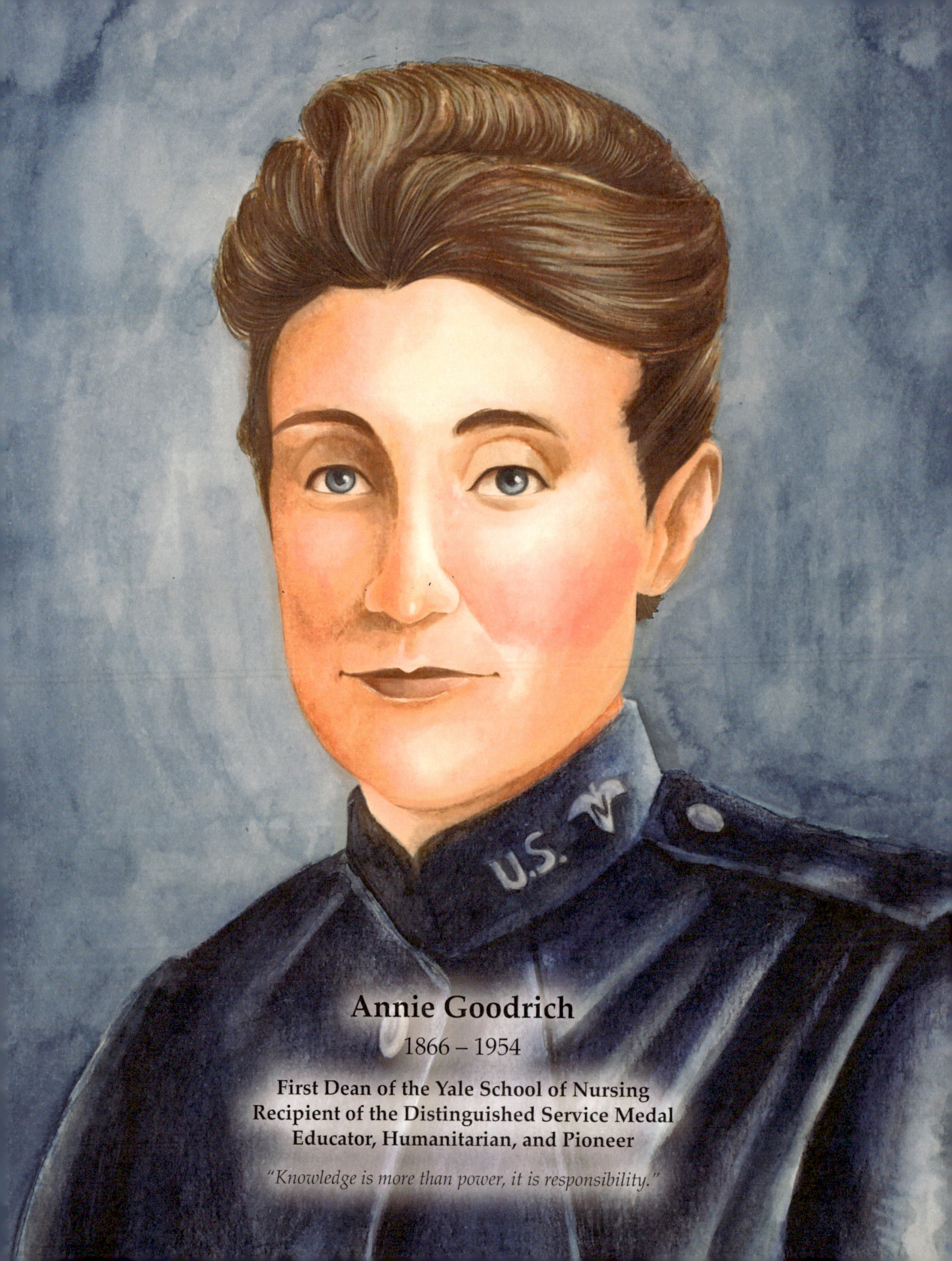

Annie Goodrich

1866 – 1954

**First Dean of the Yale School of Nursing
Recipient of the Distinguished Service Medal
Educator, Humanitarian, and Pioneer**

"Knowledge is more than power, it is responsibility."

Annie Warburton Goodrich was born on February 6, 1866, in Brunswick, New Jersey. She was the second of eight children born to Samuel and Annie Butler Goodrich. Annie's ancestors were influential. A relative named Charles Chauncy was the second president of Harvard University, and her maternal grandfather, Dr. John Butler, was a leader in the field of psychiatry. He promoted the need for compassionate care for those with mental illnesses. Annie and her siblings were fortunate to receive an excellent education. She had private tutors when she was young, and she completed high school in England when her father was sent to supervise a branch of the Equitable Life Insurance Company.

Annie's family returned to Hartford, Connecticut, to care for her ailing maternal grandparents. Annie was devoted to her grandfather and was alarmed when she observed the poor nursing care he received from a nurse whom her mother had hired to care for him. Annie decided that it was not enough to be nice and have a desire to be helpful in order to be a nurse. She believed that a nurse needed to be scientifically informed, technically knowledgeable, and relationally competent. She enrolled in the New York City Hospital School of Nursing and graduated in 1892. While she was a student, Annie and two assistants had to deal with a smallpox outbreak in the men's ward, which was where they were working. Smallpox was a contagious virus that caused fever and a disfiguring rash. As a result of a vaccine, smallpox was eliminated as a disease in 1977. Annie and her assistants had to be isolated in the ward with the patients while taking care of them. For the excellent care they provided, the hospital gave them $50.

In 1902, the majority of women who identified themselves as nurses had no formal education, similar to the young woman who had been hired to take care of Annie's grandfather. In 1913, Nurse Goodrich established standards for nursing education. She insisted that each applicant needed to have successfully completed 4 years of high school to prepare them for the 3 years of nurse training. She also required that the nursing schools undergo inspections to ensure that the students had the necessary books, equipment, and space to learn. She also proposed that there be mandatory state registration so that records were being kept to make sure that the nurses had the proper qualifications to care for patients.

Nurse Goodrich was recruited to become an assistant professor of nursing education at Teachers College, Columbia University. She was a natural teacher and demonstrated how to care for patients in the wards. She shared her wisdom and demonstrated how to provide emotional care to patients who were afraid, worried, or sad.

Nurse Goodrich served as President of the American Nurses Association in 1916 while working as the director of the Henry Street Settlement. She advocated for all nurses to receive education in preventive health and improved the salaries and working hours of the nurses at Henry Street.

When World War I broke out, there was a need for more nurses to meet all emergencies. Nurse Goodrich developed a plan to educate 1,600 nurses after being appointed as the Dean of the Army School of Nursing. This experience prepared her to be the founding dean of the Yale School of Nursing in 1933.

Society should thank Annie Warburton Goodrich for her dedication to the establishment of standards for the nursing profession. She wanted to make sure that every patient was receiving care from a nurse who was educated and highly skilled, which was also the care she wished her beloved grandfather had received when he was ill.

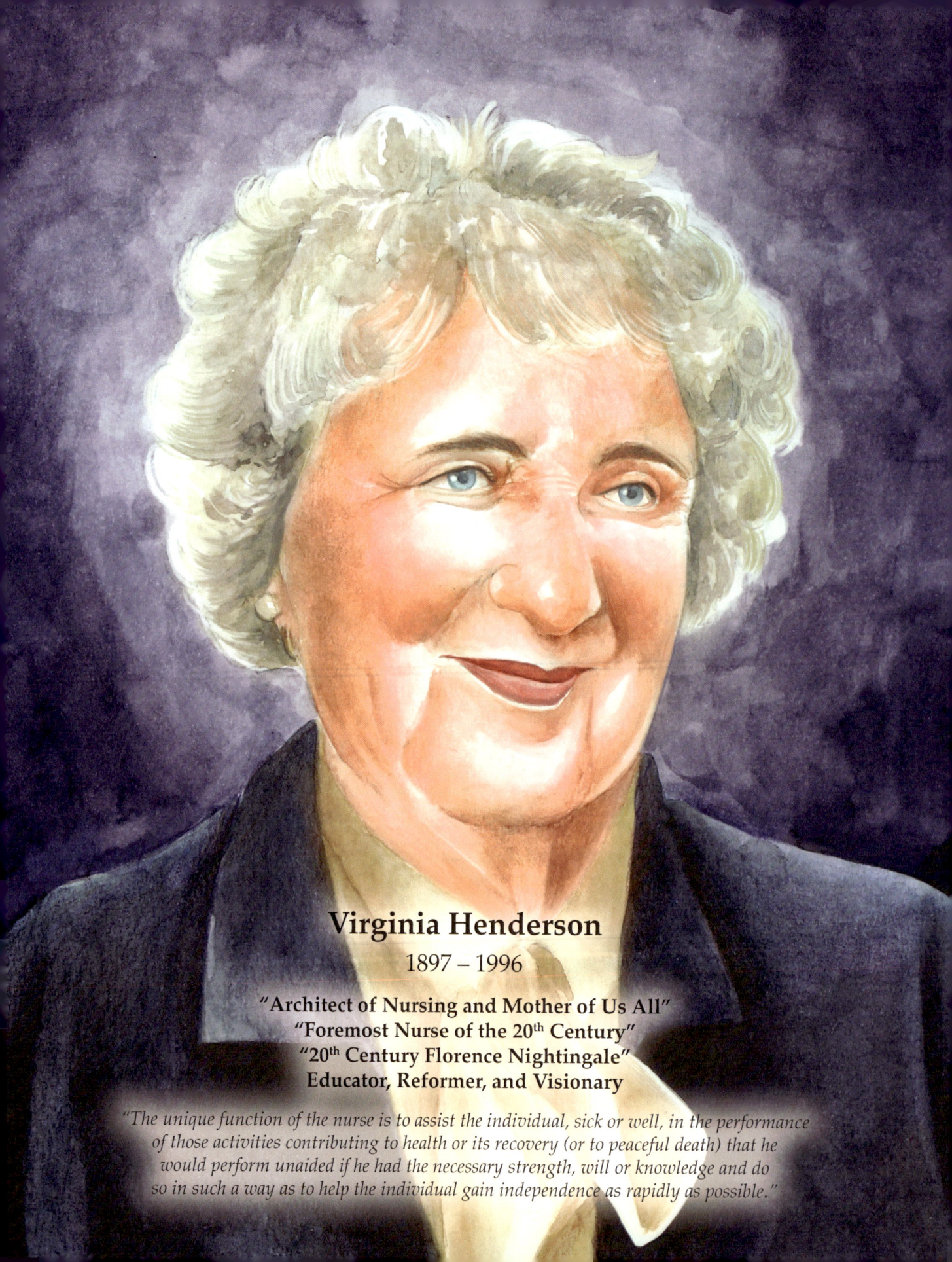

Virginia Henderson

1897 – 1996

"Architect of Nursing and Mother of Us All"
"Foremost Nurse of the 20th Century"
"20th Century Florence Nightingale"
Educator, Reformer, and Visionary

"The unique function of the nurse is to assist the individual, sick or well, in the performance of those activities contributing to health or its recovery (or to peaceful death) that he would perform unaided if he had the necessary strength, will or knowledge and do so in such a way as to help the individual gain independence as rapidly as possible."

Virginia Avenel Henderson was born in Kansas City, Missouri, on November 30, 1897, and was the fifth of eight children. Her father was an attorney who represented American Indians in lawsuits against the US government. She moved to Virginia at the age of 4; she and her sister attended a boy's preparatory school owned by their grandfather. After graduating from high school, she enlisted in the US Army School of Nursing and graduated in 1921.

After graduating, she worked as a nurse at Henry Street Settlement, founded by another nurse named Lillian Wald, on the lower east side of New York City. Many immigrants and lower-income families lived in this area. Because of tight living conditions, the citizens had poor health and a lower quality of living. The Henry Street Settlement slowly became an important place, turning its buildings into health clinics, schools, performing arts centers, and public housing. Working at Henry Street allowed Virginia the opportunity to think about delivering nursing care outside of the hospital

In 1924, Virginia became the first and only teacher at the Norfolk Protestant Hospital. After several years teaching, she decided she needed additional education. She received a bachelor's degree in nursing in 1932 and a master's degree in 1934 from Teachers College, Columbia University. She then joined the nursing faculty at Teachers College. She became a favorite teacher, as her reputation as a thinker, advocate, and reformer was becoming well known. Nurse Henderson shared her ideas about nursing: the importance of helping patients stay well and the activities they could do to recover quickly. She advocated for nurses to help patients have a peaceful death, and she noted the importance of empowering patients to be independent. She educated students on using science and stressed that the nurse's responsibility was to the patient. She provided examples of quality patient care when the doctors, nurses, pharmacists, social workers, and dietitians work together with patients and families. Virginia inspired nurses to consider the impact their care had on a person's overall health. She emphasized that nurses were the visitors in the patient-family relationship and taught nurses to include the family in care. She also taught nurses to record their observations so that doctors would know what was happening with the patient.

Nurse Henderson revised the textbook written by Bertha Hammer. The 5th edition of the *Textbook of the Principles and Practice of Nursing* was published in 1955. It was used in nursing schools worldwide to standardize education of nurses.

Nurse Henderson joined the Yale School of Nursing faculty in 1953 and discovered that most research was about the nurse, not nursing care of patients. She believed there should be more studies on the effect of nursing care on a patient's ability to get well and die with dignity. In 1972, Henderson collected all published nursing studies and assembled them in 4 volumes. This work took 12 years to complete and was one of her most important contributions. When Henderson was 75 years old, she published the 6th edition of the *Textbook of the Principles and Practice of Nursing*. She wrote the book so any person could grasp how to take care of a relative or friend.

Throughout her career, Nurse Henderson promoted nursing and nursing research to improve care of patients. She believed that nurses needed to be educated to think, use research to guide decisions, and partner with patients so that they could recover or die peacefully. She redefined nursing practice and influenced generations of nurses through her teachings and writings. Virginia lived to be 98 and witnessed her dreams for nursing practice be adopted by nurses throughout the world.

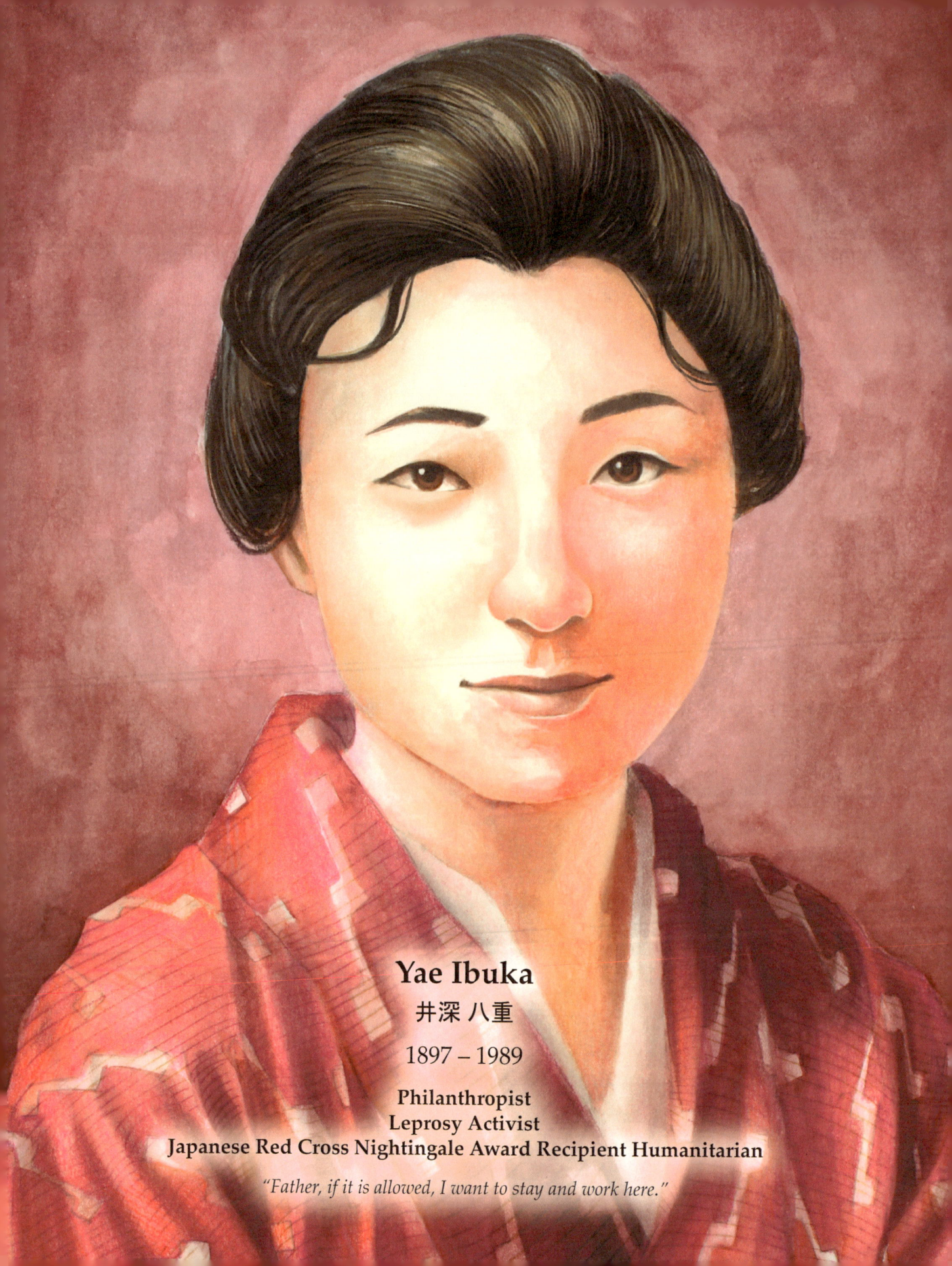

Yae Ibuka

井深 八重

1897 – 1989

Philanthropist
Leprosy Activist
Japanese Red Cross Nightingale Award Recipient Humanitarian

"Father, if it is allowed, I want to stay and work here."

Yae Ibuka was born on October 23, 1897, in Taipei, Formosa, now known as Taipei, Taiwan. She was the daughter of Hikosabura Ibuka, a congressman. Little is known about Yae's mother. Due to her social status, Yae led a privileged childhood.

She graduated from Doshisa Women's College in 1919 and began teaching English to school children in Nagasaki, Japan. At 22 years of age, Yae began to feel unwell and noticed that she was developing lumps and bumps on her arms and legs that were not going away. She was diagnosed with leprosy, also known as Hansen's Disease. Hansen's disease is caused by a slow-growing bacteria that can lead to crippling of the hands and feet, paralysis, and blindness. There was no treatment or cure when Yae was diagnosed. People were treated as outcasts and were sent to live in "leper colonies." Yae was admitted to Koyama Fukusei Hospital, the oldest hospital for lepers in Japan, and remained there for 3 years.

After spending years in the hospital and realizing that she was not getting better, she traveled to Tokyo to seek another opinion and get an explanation about her condition. The doctor told her that she did not have leprosy and had been misdiagnosed. Yae had spent 3 years living in a hospital needlessly and had observed many things while being a patient. She was grateful for the loving kindness that Father Drouart de Lézey, the director of the hospital, had showed to each patient. She watched in awe as he listened to the patients and comforted them on his daily rounds. Yae became convinced that her calling was to care for people with leprosy by becoming a nurse. She was determined to make a difference in the lives of others, most significantly those with leprosy. In 1923, she accomplished her goal and began working at the Koyama Fukusei Hospital, where she had been a patient. At the time, she was the only qualified nurse caring for patients in the hospital.

Nurse Ibuka worked at Koyama Fukusei Hospital for many years, eventually becoming the chief nurse. She was beloved by her patients, as she was able to understand their pain, suffering, and feelings of isolation. She was known to use her own money to help her patients and their families. Yae earned the title of "honorary mother" by many.

Nurse Ibuka's work earned her many awards. In 1959, she received a special honor from Pope John Paul XXIII, the Pontifical Order of St. Sylvester. In 1961, the Japanese Red Cross awarded Yae with the Florence Nightingale medal. The Florence Nightingale medal, created in 1912, is the highest international distinction a nurse can achieve and is given to nurses for "exceptional courage and devotion to the wounded, sick or disabled or to civilian victims of a conflict or disaster or exemplary services or a creative and pioneering spirit in the areas of public health or nursing education."

Yae also invested her time and energy in advancing nursing practice and education in Japan. She became the first president of the Japan Catholic Nurses Association and remained the chief nurse at Koyama Fukusei Hospital until 1978, when she retired.

Nurse Yae Ibuka died in 1989 at her cherished Koyama Fukusei Hospital, one day before its 100th anniversary. At the anniversary celebration, she was honored for her dedication with a special award that was given by Princess Takamatsu (Kikuko) of Japan.

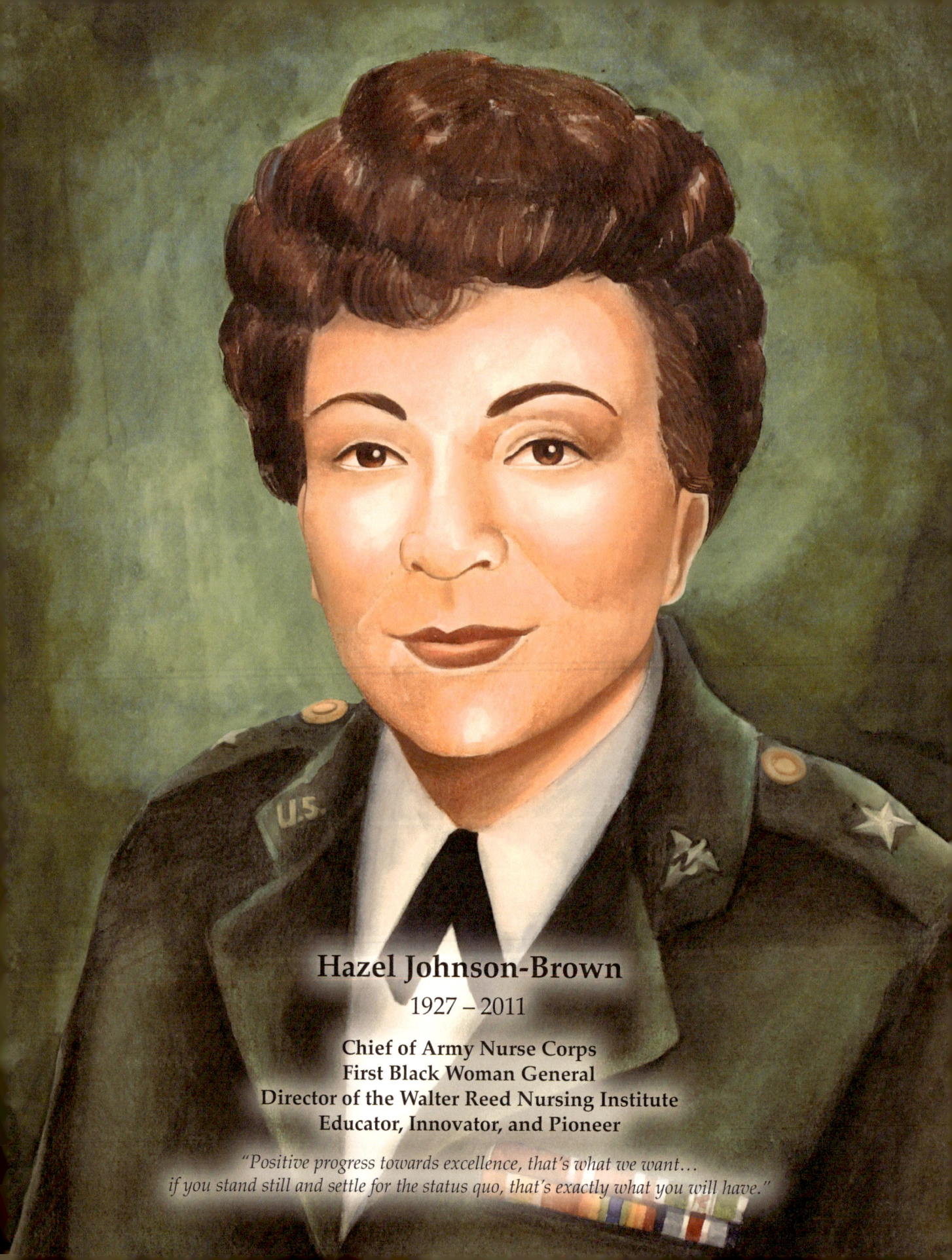

Hazel Johnson-Brown

1927 – 2011

Chief of Army Nurse Corps
First Black Woman General
Director of the Walter Reed Nursing Institute
Educator, Innovator, and Pioneer

"Positive progress towards excellence, that's what we want...
if you stand still and settle for the status quo, that's exactly what you will have."

Hazel Winifred Johnson was born in 1927 in West Chester, Pennsylvania, to Garnett Henley and Clarence L. Johnson, Sr. Hazel was one of seven children. Her parents were farmers, and they lived off the land, growing fruits and vegetables and raising livestock. They instilled in their children the values of discipline, respect, and hard work. Hazel was inspired to become a nurse at the age of twelve after interacting with "Miss Fritz," a public health nurse who would visit the family and check on their health and well-being.

She applied to nursing school after graduating from high school but was denied admission. Hazel was told that "they have never and would never" accept a black woman into their program. Determined to be a nurse, she applied to other schools, eventually moving to New York City to attend the Harlem School of Nursing. After graduating from her nursing program in 1950, she began her career in the emergency department at Harlem Hospital. After three years, she returned to her home state of Pennsylvania and began working at the Philadelphia Veteran's Administration (VA) Hospital, caring for patients with heart disease. She was promoted to Head Nurse within three months. She enrolled in the nursing program at Villanova University to earn her bachelor's degree and began thinking about joining the Army so she could travel and explore the opportunities the Army could offer.

Hazel enlisted in the Army and worked at Walter Reed Medical Center in Washington, DC. and the 8,169th Hospital in Camp Zama, Japan. In 1957, Nurse Johnson left the Army and returned to civilian life, resuming her studies at Villanova University and rejoining the staff at Philadelphia VA. In 1958, she entered the Army Nurse Corp's Registered Nurse Student Program so that she could receive financial assistance for her education. She specialized in operating room nursing and was to be sent to Vietnam, but a lung infection prevented her from being deployed. The nurse who replaced her was killed in a missile attack on the hospital, and several others were killed or injured, as well. Hazel was sent overseas again to become the Chief Nurse at the largest branch of the U.S. Army in South Korea.

Hazel developed a reputation for being smart, respectful, and extremely organized. During her time in the military, Hazel accomplished many things. She increased the opportunities for Reserve Officer Training Corps (ROTC) nursing students to receive academic scholarships. She created nursing practice standards, developed a new sterilizing process for field hospitals, and encouraged nurses to conduct research and publish their results. She furthered her own education by earning a master's degree from Columbia University and a doctoral degree from The Catholic University of America.

President Jimmy Carter nominated her to become the Chief of the Army Nurse Corps in 1979, and with the promotion, she received the new rank of Brigadier General. Hazel Johnson became the first black woman general and the first Chief of the Army Nurse Corp with a PhD. Hazel's parents did not live long enough to witness this historic moment. Her mother died a day before her promotion was announced. In 1981, Hazel married David Brown and hyphenated her name. They divorced a few years later.

Always a planner, General Johnson-Brown knew that she wanted to remain active in retirement. She joined the nursing faculty at Georgetown University. She was also recruited by the American Nurses Association to lead the government relations unit. She designed the Center for Health Policy at George Mason University, which educated nurses about healthcare policy.

Hazel hoped to be remembered as a good person who did her best. She succeeded!

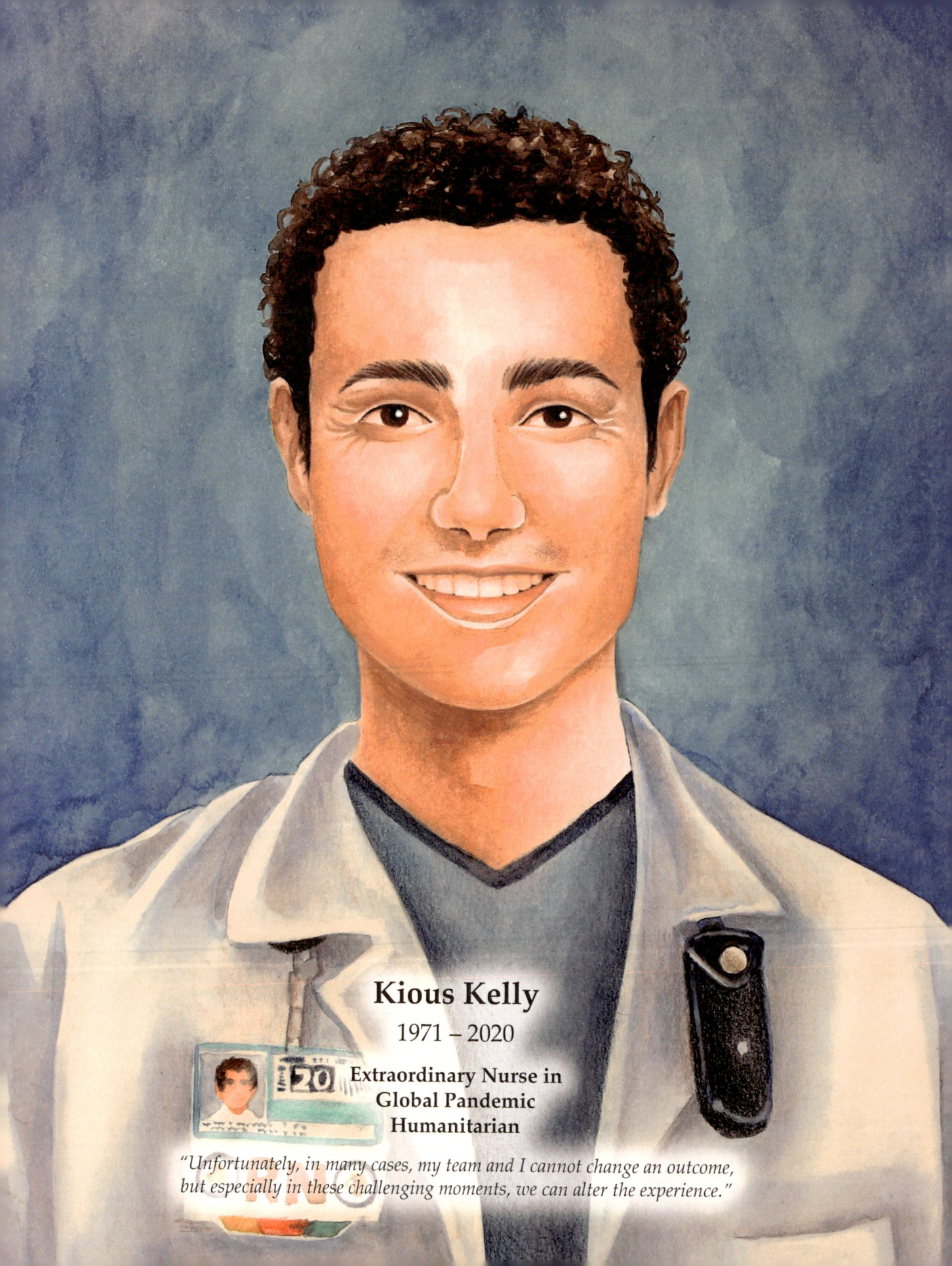

Kious Kelly

1971 – 2020

**Extraordinary Nurse in
Global Pandemic
Humanitarian**

*"Unfortunately, in many cases, my team and I cannot change an outcome,
but especially in these challenging moments, we can alter the experience."*

Kious Kelly was the oldest of two children and was born on September 28, 1971, to Karen Kious and Marion Smith. He grew up in Lansing, Michigan, with his sister, Marya, and excelled in the arts, acting in every school play in high school. He was awarded an academic scholarship and was unsure whether he should study engineering or dance. His father advised him to study engineering, but he followed his passion and became a dancer. His birth certificate listed his name as Marion James Smith, IV. As an adult, he legally changed his name to Kious Jordan Kelly, which was a family name.

Kious studied ballet at Butler University in Indianapolis and then moved to New York City. After dancing with several New York ballet companies, Kious wanted to make a career change. He decided that he could use his creative talents to ease the suffering of others and enrolled in the nursing program at New York University. Upon graduation in 2012, Kious joined the staff at Mount Sinai West in Manhattan.

Nurse Kelly brought his joyful disposition, generosity of spirit, and passion for learning to the bedside. He was dedicated to helping his patients heal, not just recover, from an illness. Kious was aware of the burdens many patients carried in daily life and was committed to helping them. He encountered a gentleman who did not want to be discharged from the hospital because it was winter and he was homeless and had no coat. Kious gave the man his own coat. He purchased items for patients with his own money so that they had the items they needed in order to be able to use their medical equipment correctly. He would check in at homeless shelters to see if he could provide nursing care to individuals who might need healthcare. He gave patients his personal phone number and encouraged them to call, as he lived close to the hospital.

Kious was promoted to assistant nurse manager. In this leadership role, Nurse Kelly guided nurses in providing high-quality patient care, ensured that there were enough nurses each shift to give safe care, and created an environment where nurses could thrive. Kious was respected by his staff, and the nurses regularly sought him out for his opinion.

In March of 2020, New York City hospitals became overwhelmed with patients infected with COVID-19 who were seeking life-saving care. COVID-19, a highly contagious infectious virus for which there is no treatment or cure, was stretching the resources of hospitals, nursing homes, and emergency medical services. Thousands of infected people were going to Emergency Rooms with coughs and high fevers. They were struggling to breathe and were exhausted. Patients' conditions changed very quickly, and they often needed to be transferred to the Intensive Care Unit (ICU), where they needed to have a breathing tube inserted and were then placed on a machine to help them breathe.

The nurses, doctors, and respiratory therapists caring for people infected with COVID-19 have to wear special clothing called "personal protective equipment" (PPE). Each time a nurse, doctor, or other caregiver entered the room of a patient with COVID-19, they had to wear a mask, face shield, gown, and gloves to protect themselves from becoming infected. Nurse Kelly made sure that every caregiver entering a patient's room was wearing the equipment correctly. He wanted to keep them safe.

Kious Jordan Kelly died on March 24, 2020, six days after becoming infected with COVID-19. Kious is one of hundreds of frontline caregivers who have died while caring for the people suffering and dying from COVID-19. Kious loved being a nurse, and his patients and colleagues loved him back.

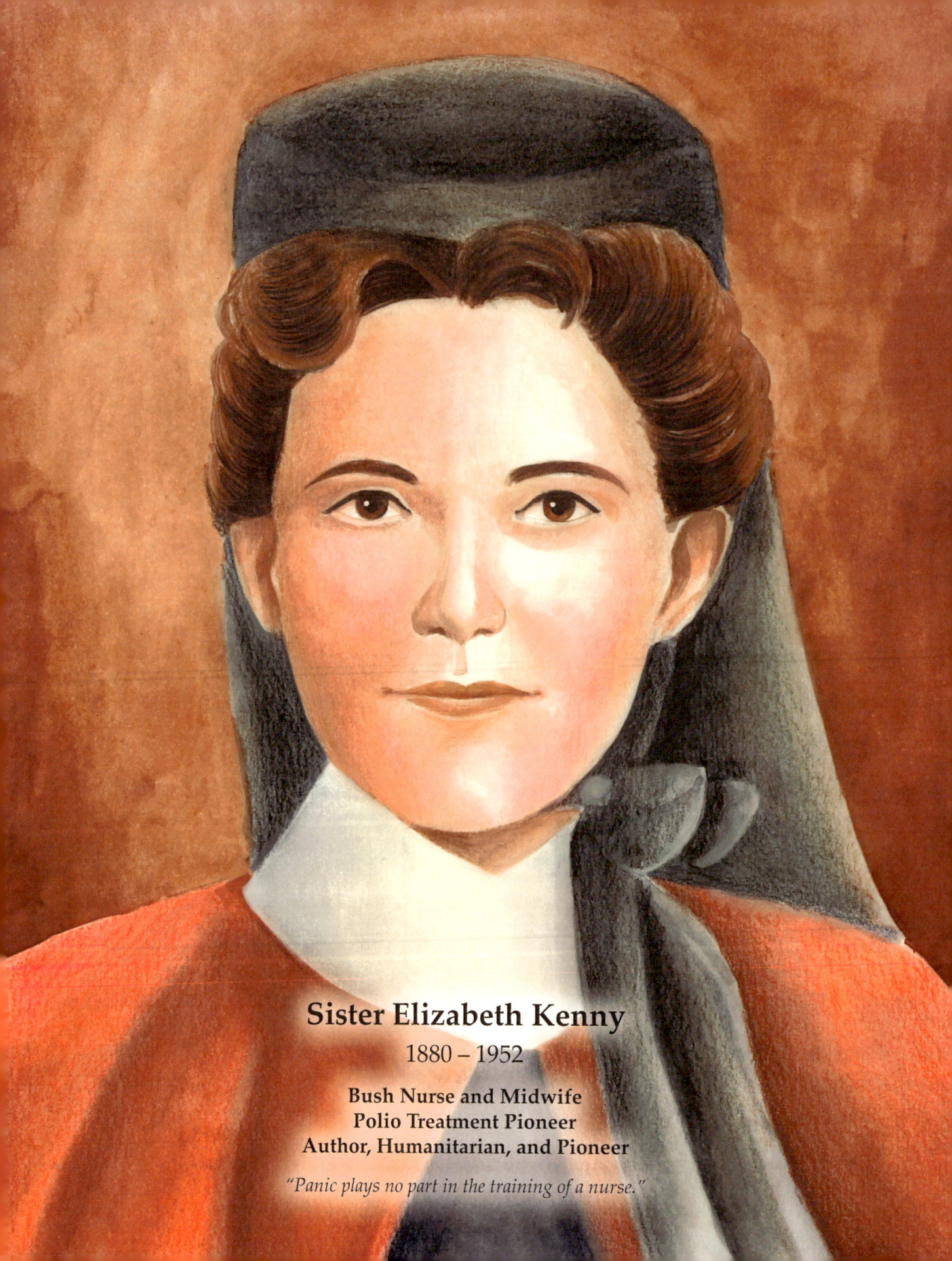

Sister Elizabeth Kenny

1880 – 1952

Bush Nurse and Midwife
Polio Treatment Pioneer
Author, Humanitarian, and Pioneer

"Panic plays no part in the training of a nurse."

Elizabeth Kenny was born in New South Wales, a state on the east coast of Australia, in 1880. Her parents were farmers, and she was homeschooled by her mother for many years. When Elizabeth was 17, she broke her wrist while riding her horse, and her father took her to visit a doctor for treatment. While being treated, Elizabeth's interest in medicine, the human body, and how muscles worked was sparked; she studied the doctor's anatomy books and model skeleton. Although she was interested in medicine, it was not a career that was approved for young women in the 1800s in Australia, so she became a religion and music teacher.

In 1907, Elizabeth, who was called Lisa by her family, changed careers and began working in the kitchen at a local midwives' cottage, where she learned about midwifery by paying attention to the work others were completing. She had a local seamstress make her a nurse uniform, and she returned to her home state and began offering her services as a bush nurse. In Australia, bush nurses were nurses who offered their services to people living in remote areas, who didn't have easy access to doctors and hospitals. Bush nurses delivered babies, delivered first aid care, and helped educate people about hygiene and safety. As a bush nurse, Elizabeth opened a small hospital. She helped deliver babies and treat children who suffered from polio by using the information she remembered from the doctor's anatomy books and model skeleton. Polio is a disease that can lead to paralysis due to contracted or stiff muscles. Elizabeth treated Polio afflicted patients by wrapping their legs with hot compresses made from blankets.

After working as a bush nurse, she did her part to help Australia and England during World War I by working on cargo ships that carried soldiers and supplies to and from Australia and England. Although she was not an officially qualified nurse, nurses were needed for these missions. She made sixteen trips and earned the title "Sister" from the Australian Army Nursing Corps. This title designated her as a highly qualified nurse. After her service, she was honorably discharged and returned home to care for victims of the 1918 Spanish Flu epidemic.

While caring for patients during the epidemic, Sister Kenny also cared for her elderly mother and her neighbors. One neighbor, a girl named Sylvia, was trampled by a horse. When brought to Sister Kenny, she made a stretcher from a door and helped transport Sylvia to a local doctor. This stretcher was so helpful in keeping Sylvia safe and transporting her, that Sister Kenny made several more stretchers and gave them to local ambulance services, calling the invention the "Sylvia Stretcher."

After traveling around Australia to sell the Sylvia Stretcher, Sister Kenny used her talents and skills to treat children with polio. She set up a polio treatment facility and helped so many children regain the ability to walk by using her methods of special exercises and hot compresses that she was able to open several other clinics in other cities across Australia, England, and America, and she published a book about her methods and successes in 1943.

Her work faced some criticism from doctors who disagreed with her methods, but when they saw the effects and successes she had in treatment, they changed their minds and no longer doubted her.

Sister Kenny continued her work with people recovering from polio across the world until her death, which was caused by complications from Parkinson's disease, in 1952. Her funeral was broadcast across Australia and in parts of the United States.

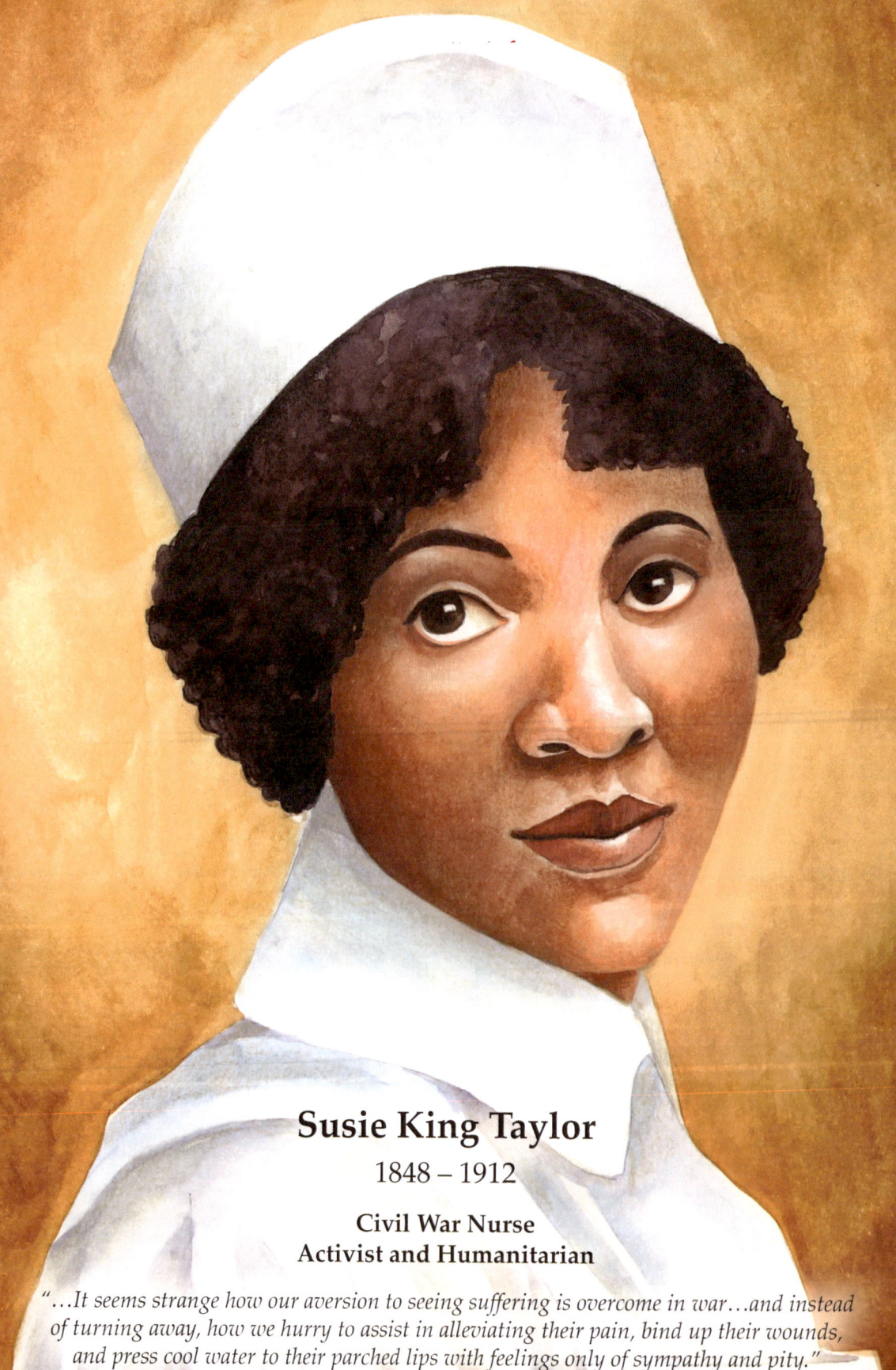

Susie King Taylor

1848 – 1912

Civil War Nurse
Activist and Humanitarian

"…It seems strange how our aversion to seeing suffering is overcome in war…and instead of turning away, how we hurry to assist in alleviating their pain, bind up their wounds, and press cool water to their parched lips with feelings only of sympathy and pity."

Susan Ann Baker was born into slavery on August 6, 1848, on the Grest Plantation in Liberty County, Georgia. She was the eldest of nine children who were born to Hagar Ann Reed and Raymond Baker. The Grests, the plantation owners, had no children of their own and were loving and kind to the Baker children. At age 7, Susie was permitted to go live with her grandmother, a freed slave, in Savannah, Georgia. Despite Georgia law prohibiting the education of African Americans, her grandmother, Dolly, was determined that Susie would learn how to read and write, and she sent her to two secret schools run by free African American women. She learned the basics and was further instructed by two white youths.

The Civil War had begun when South Carolina became the first state to secede from the Union. In 1862, Taylor and an uncle were able to escape slavery by fleeing to a federal gunboat called the U.S.S. Potomska, which was near Confederate-held Fort Pulaski. They, along with hundreds of other African Americans fleeing slavery, went to live on St. Simons Island, occupied by Union forces, off the coast of Georgia.

Union officers noted Susie's education, and they asked her to form a school for the many freed slave children. She became the first African American teacher at the age of 14, and she taught 40 children in day school and many adults at night.

Susie moved to Beaufort, South Carolina, where the 1st South Carolina Volunteer Infantry Regiment was camped. Later named the 33rd US Colored Infantry Regiment, it was one of the first African American military units. Susie married Edward King, a sergeant in the unit, and traveled with the unit for 4 years.

Susie was enlisted to be the laundress, but it became obvious to the unit commander that Susie had much to contribute. She maintained guns, taught soldiers how to read and write, and nursed the wounded. Susie worked alongside Clara Barton, tending to the soldiers. The Union soldiers were impressed with her compassion, knowledge, and courage. Like most Civil War nurses, she did not go to school to learn how to be a nurse. She used a combination of traditional and folk remedies. Her grandmother was a healer and used plants, roots, and tree bark to make medicines. She taught her granddaughter about sassafras tea, which Susie drank daily. Susie believed the tea prevented her from contracting any of the diseases common in camp, such as cholera, diarrhea, malaria, measles, pneumonia, and typhoid. She had received the smallpox vaccine as a child and fearlessly tended to those who suffered with it.

When the war was over, Susie and her husband, Edward, moved to Savannah, where she opened a private school for African American children. Edward died suddenly before their first child was born. Susie lost her income when public schools opened, and became a domestic servant to a wealthy family. She moved with them to Boston, where she met and married Russell Taylor.

Even though Susie no longer worked as a nurse, she still loved nursing. She served with the Women's Relief Corps and helped champion the Army Nurse Pension Act of 1892, which provided assistance to soldiers and hospitals. Susie wrote of her wartime experiences in the book *Reminiscences of My Life in Camp With the 33rd United States Colored Troops Late 1st S.C. Volunteers*, which was published in 1902. She was the first black woman to publish a Civil War memoir.

Susie King Taylor never received a military pension or recognition for her service, as she had been classified as a laundress, not a nurse.

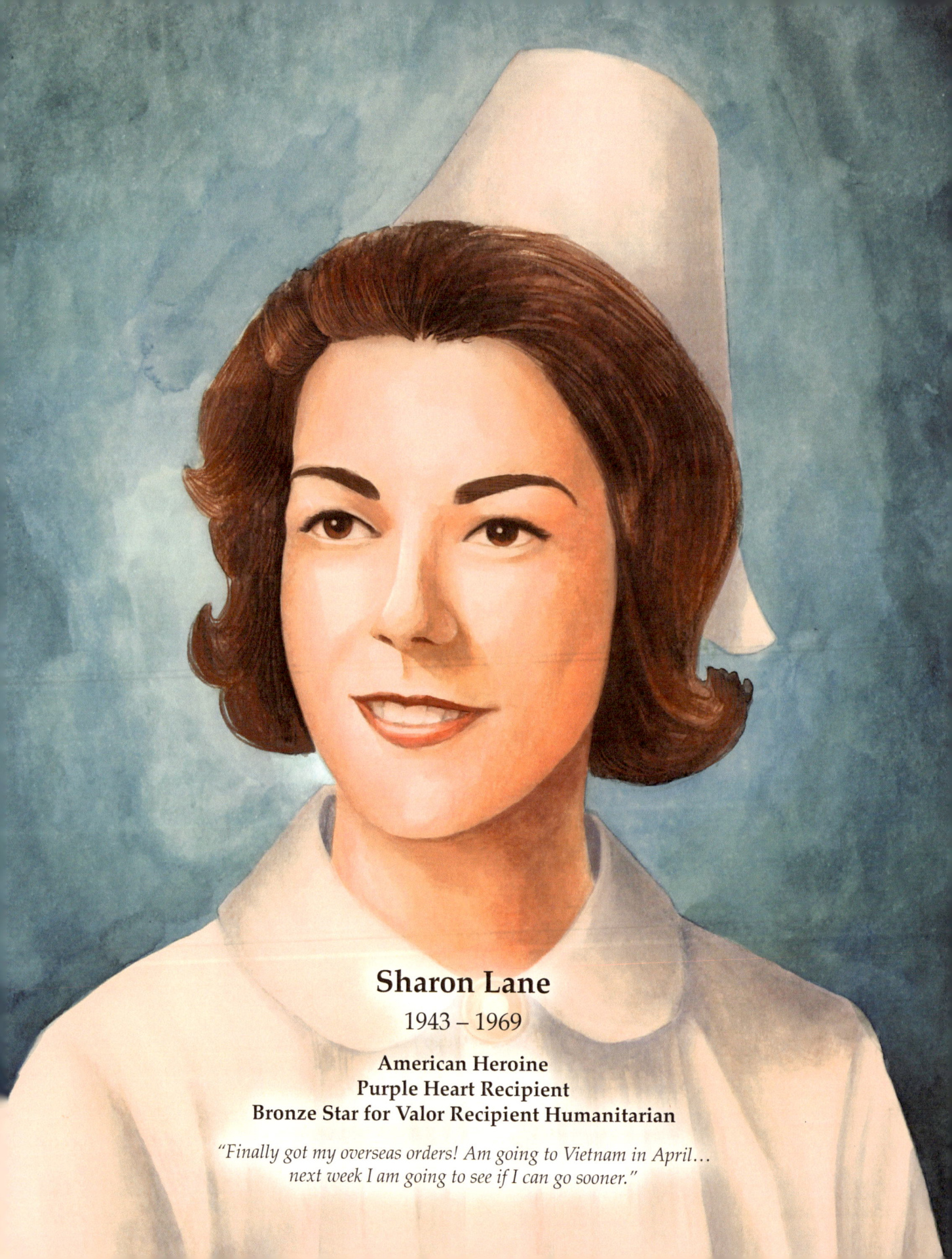

Sharon Lane

1943 – 1969

American Heroine
Purple Heart Recipient
Bronze Star for Valor Recipient Humanitarian

"Finally got my overseas orders! Am going to Vietnam in April…
next week I am going to see if I can go sooner."

Sharon Ann Lane was born on July 7, 1943, in Zanesville, Ohio. She was the middle of three children born to John and Kay Lane. Sharon was quiet and fun loving, and she enjoyed listening to the music of Elvis Presley, Paul Anka, and Fabian as a teenager in the 1950s. While many business schools tried to recruit her, assuring her that working as a secretary would provide a very fulfilling life, Sharon chose to become a nurse.

While in her first year at Aultman School of Nursing in Canton, Ohio, Sharon smuggled a dead frog out of the class so that she could repeat the dissection and label all of the organs in order to prepare for an upcoming exam. To preserve the frog for future study, she stored it on the windowsill of her dorm room, not really thinking about the warm air coming through the window! Sharon graduated in 1965 and began working on a maternity unit at Aultman Hospital. She left nursing after two years and enrolled in business school, but she did not find the work satisfying. Sharon returned to nursing and joined the U.S. Army Nurse Corps Reserve in 1968.

Nurse Lane completed basic training at Fort Sam Houston Army Base in Houston, Texas, and was assigned to the Fitzsimmons General Hospital in Denver, Colorado, to begin her career as an Army nurse. She cared for patients with tuberculosis, which is a bacterial infection that affects the lungs and can also spread to the spine and the brain. After being promoted to 1st Lieutenant, Nurse Lane was transferred to the Intensive Care Unit (ICU). She cared for critically ill patients until she received orders to Vietnam.

Sharon was assigned to the 312th Evacuation Chu Lai in Vietnam. Her first day was only a six -hour shift so she could become familiar with the hospital and adjust to the time change. Sharon worked on the unit dedicated to caring for Vietnamese patients. The unit was challenging because of the language barrier and the fears of her patients, who had never before received medical care. 1st Lieutenant Lane worked 60 hours a week and spent her days off caring for critically ill American soldiers in the ICU.

First Lieutenant Lane had just finished her rounds on the morning of June 8, 1969, checking on the 26 patients on her unit. Sharon had been in Vietnam just six weeks and had volunteered to work the night shift. There had been reports that the North Vietnamese were planning an attack, so everyone working that night wore flak vests, a form of body armor, to protect them from shrapnel. The vests were big and bulky, and as the shift progressed and there were no attacks, the staff took them off. As the sun was rising, the quiet of the early morning was shattered by a rocket blast that left her ward in ruin. Sharon died instantly from shrapnel that pierced her chest while she was trying to move patients to safety. She was 25 years old.

Sharon was smart, dedicated, and compassionate. She had planned to re-enlist in the Army because she found her work rewarding and hoped to see the world. She was the only nurse serving in Vietnam who was killed by enemy fire. After her death, she was awarded the Purple Heart, the Bronze Star, and the National Order of Vietnam Medal, which was awarded by the Vietnamese government.

First Lieutenant Sharon Ann Lane's name is carved into the Vietnam War Memorial, along with 58,299 others, 8 of whom are women. Her name can be found on Panel W23, Line 112.

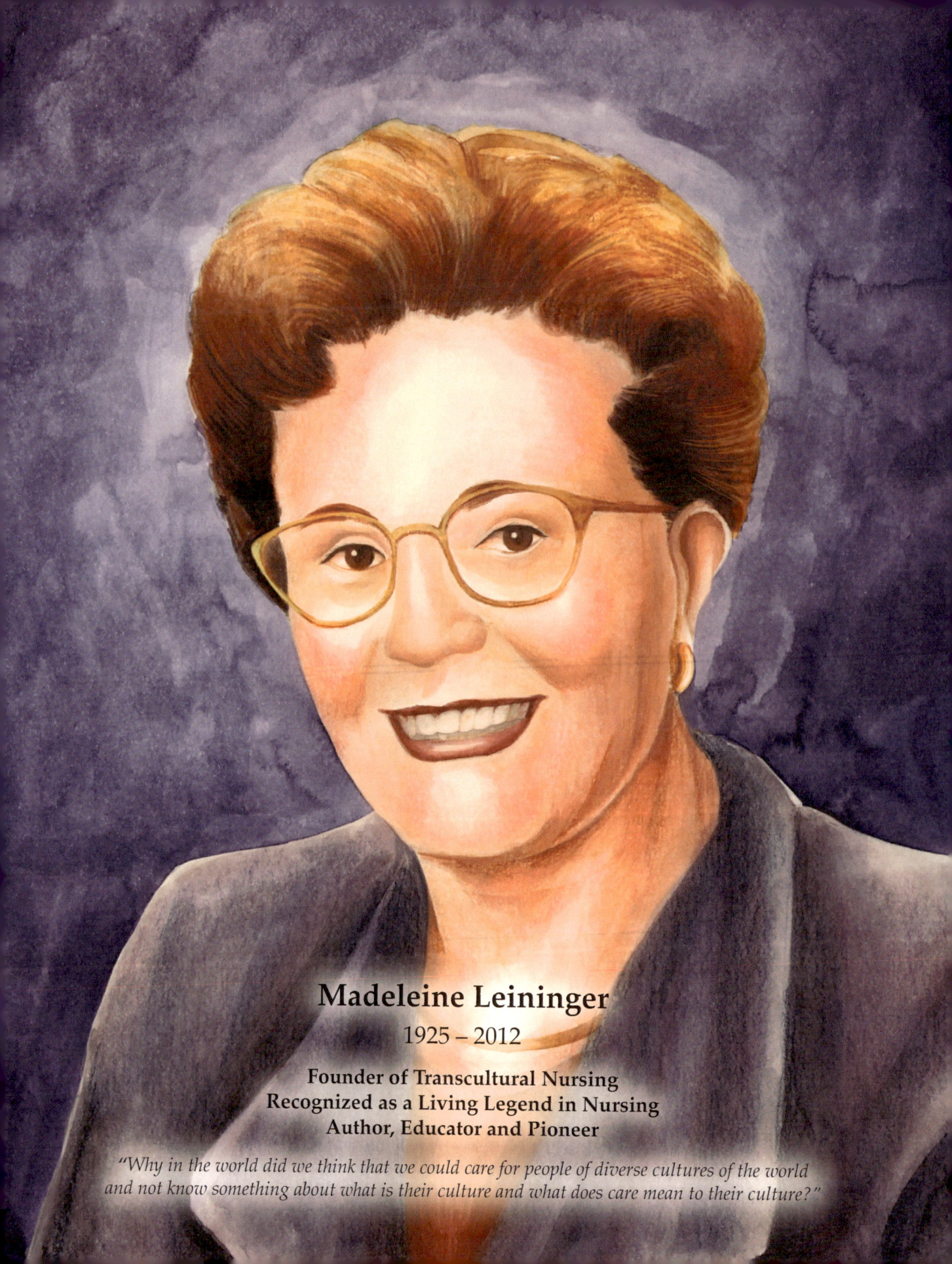

Madeleine Leininger

1925 – 2012

**Founder of Transcultural Nursing
Recognized as a Living Legend in Nursing
Author, Educator and Pioneer**

*"Why in the world did we think that we could care for people of diverse cultures of the world
and not know something about what is their culture and what does care mean to their culture?"*

Madeleine Leininger was born on a farm on July 13, 1925, in Sutton, Nebraska. She was the middle of five children born to George and Irene Leininger. Her father was a farmer, and her mother was a homemaker. Madeleine was introduced to the art of nursing while caring for her beloved aunt, who suffered from heart disease. After her aunt died, her parents took in her 5 cousins, and the Leininger house was overflowing with children. Since her parents did not have money to send Madeleine to college, she entered the Cadet Nurse Corps, a government program that educated nurses to help with the nursing shortage during World War II.

Madeleine was curious about the world and continued her education, earning several degrees. She was the first nurse to earn a PhD in anthropology. Anthropology, which is the science of humanity, explores how human beings' traditions, social customs, and beliefs influence behavior.

Early in her career, Nurse Leininger worked with children in Cincinnati from diverse cultures and noticed that there was a difference in how the children responded to the treatment. While working there, she met a woman who would change the course of her life: the famed anthropologist Margaret Mead. Dr. Mead was the most celebrated anthropologist of the 20th century and made several important discoveries. Dr. Mead also encouraged women to seek careers outside of the traditional roles while championing motherhood. When Madeline asked Dr. Mead if she thought there was a connection between anthropology and nursing, she was told, "Well that is something for you to discover," and discover she did! She packed her suitcase and headed for New Guinea, a large island in the Pacific Ocean.

For two years, Nurse Leininger lived in a hut among the Gadsup people of the Eastern Highlands of New Guinea. It was the early 1960s, and upon arrival to the village, she quickly observed that there was no indoor plumbing or electricity, and there were no appliances, telephones, or modern modes of transportation. The Gadsup people had little or no contact with the western world and had never met a white, unmarried nurse researcher. Many of the villagers thought she might be a sorcerer and kept their distance. Madeleine was able to tell that she was gaining the villagers' trust when they began to give her food that was not rotten.

In the beginning of her research, Madeleine learned that there were no clocks, calendars, or written records in the village. The history of the village was passed down from generation to generation through storytelling. Over the course of her career, Nurse Leininger studied 15 unique cultures and used this knowledge to develop a theory she titled Transcultural Nursing. Her theory provides a road map nurses use to honor and respect the family roles, communication patterns, nutritional practices, spiritual beliefs, and death rituals of the patients who have cultures different from their own.

Nurse Leininger was an enthusiastic teacher, and she introduced her theory to thousands of students. She was a faculty member at the University of Cincinnati and the University of Colorado. She was also a visiting professor at universities across the world, including universities in Japan, New Zealand, Sweden, China, and Australia. She served as the Dean of Nursing at several universities, including the University of Washington and the University of Utah. She served as a Professor of Nursing and as the adjunct Professor of Anthropology at Wayne State University, and she was given an entirely new role as Director of Transcultural Nursing offerings there.

Although Madeleine traveled the world, she died in Nebraska, the state where she was born, at the age of 87.

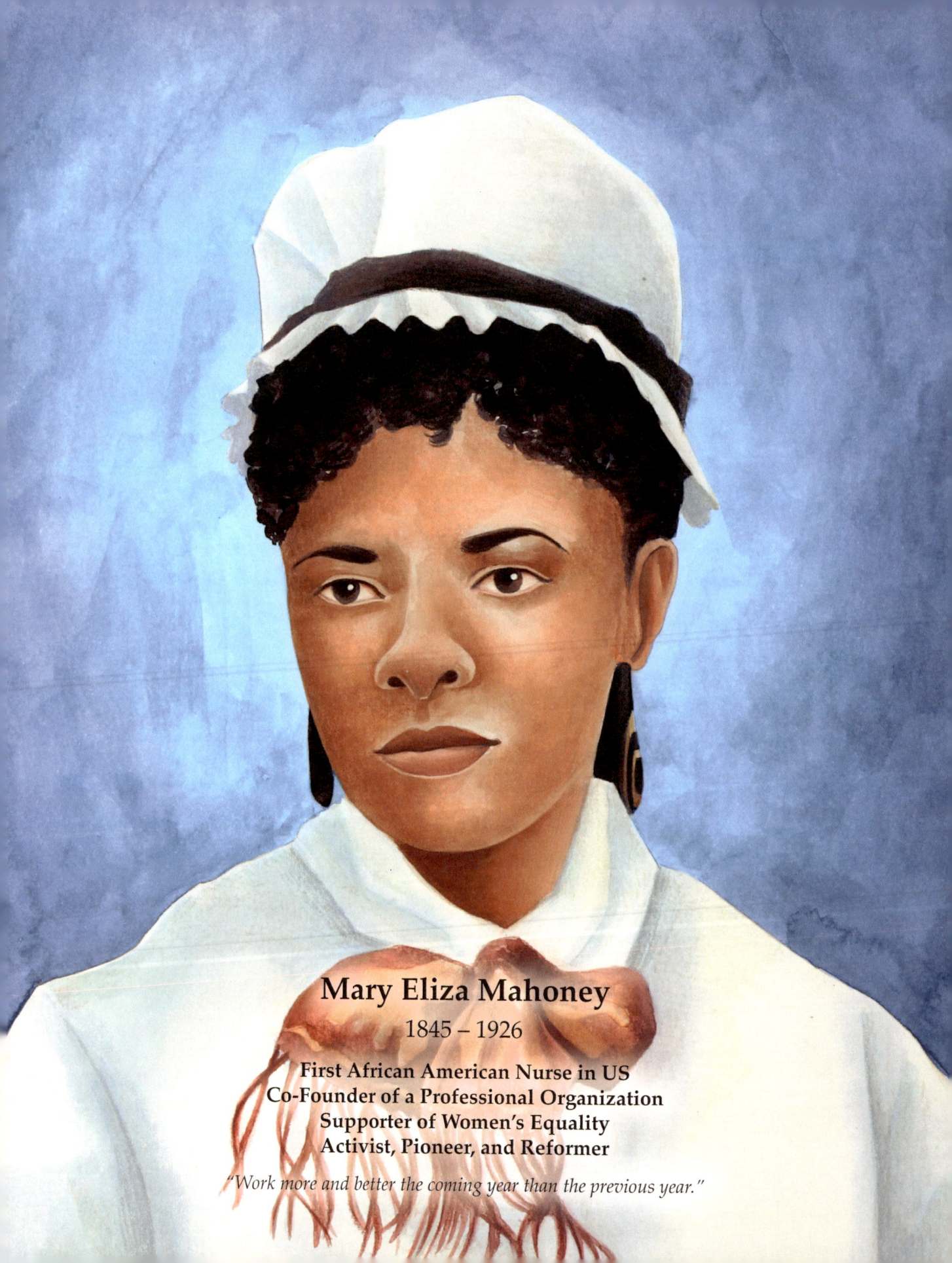

Mary Eliza Mahoney

1845 – 1926

First African American Nurse in US
Co-Founder of a Professional Organization
Supporter of Women's Equality
Activist, Pioneer, and Reformer

"Work more and better the coming year than the previous year."

Mary Eliza Mahoney was born on May 7, 1845, in Dorchester, Massachusetts, to Mary June Seward and Charles Mahoney. She was the oldest of three children. Her parents were freed slaves who had moved north before the American Civil War, in pursuit of a life with less racial discrimination.

She knew very early in her life that she wanted to be a nurse. Yet at this time, it was very unusual for African American women to be accepted into nursing schools, even in the north. Although she began to show an interest in enrolling into a nursing program at the age of 18, it was not until she was 33 years old that she was accepted into the New England Hospital for Women and Children nursing program. It may have been her dedicated work at this hospital as a cook, maid, and washerwoman that led to her acceptance into the nursing program. The training required long hours, and she worked from 6:00 a.m. to 9:00 p.m. Out of her class of 40 students, Mary and two other white women were the only ones to receive their nursing certificates. On August 1, 1879, 14 years after the end of the Civil War, she became the first black woman in the United States to become a Registered Nurse.

Following her graduation, Mary worked primarily as a private-duty nurse, as racial discrimination prevented her from working as a public nurse. She earned a distinguished reputation for her work, especially because of her dedicated care of mothers and newborns. Those who employed Mary praised her professionalism, compassion, and excellent care.

Nurse Mahoney believed that all people should have the opportunity to chase their dreams without racial discrimination. She worked tirelessly to abolish discrimination in the nursing field. Mary became one of the original members of the predominately white Nurses Associated Alumnae of the United States and Canada (NAAUSC). This organization later became the American Nurses Association (ANA), now the national organization for all Registered Nurses. Because the NAAUSC was not particularly welcoming of African American nurses, Nurse Mahoney became the co-founder of the National Association of Colored Graduate Nurses (NACGN) with two nurse colleagues. This association was dedicated to eliminating racial discrimination for all nurses. Mary was invited to give the opening speech at the first convention of the new organization. Mary, who was 5 feet tall and weighed 90 pounds, was able to use her ability to inspire and capture the attention of the attendees as she spoke about the inequalities in nursing education at the time.

Following her retirement from professional nursing, Nurse Mahoney was active in concerns related to women's equality and was a strong supporter of women's suffrage. In 1920, in Boston, she was among the first women to register to vote after the passage of the 19th Amendment on August 26, 1920.

In recognition of Mary Mahoney's outstanding example to nurses of all races, the NACGN established an award in her name. When NACGN merged with the American Nurses Association in 1951, the award was continued. Today, it is bestowed biennially, meaning it is awarded every 2 years, to outstanding nurses from minority groups.

Helen Sullivan Miller, who was awarded the Mary Mahoney Medal in 1968, decided to travel to Everett, Massachusetts, to visit Mary Mahoney's grave. Helen was unable to locate the tombstone immediately and felt that Mary deserved a proper monument. She led a fundraising effort, and the tombstone was designed by another Mahoney medal recipient named Mabel Keaton Staupers. In 2006, the United States Congress honored Mary Eliza Mahoney by declaring her the first professionally trained African American nurse.

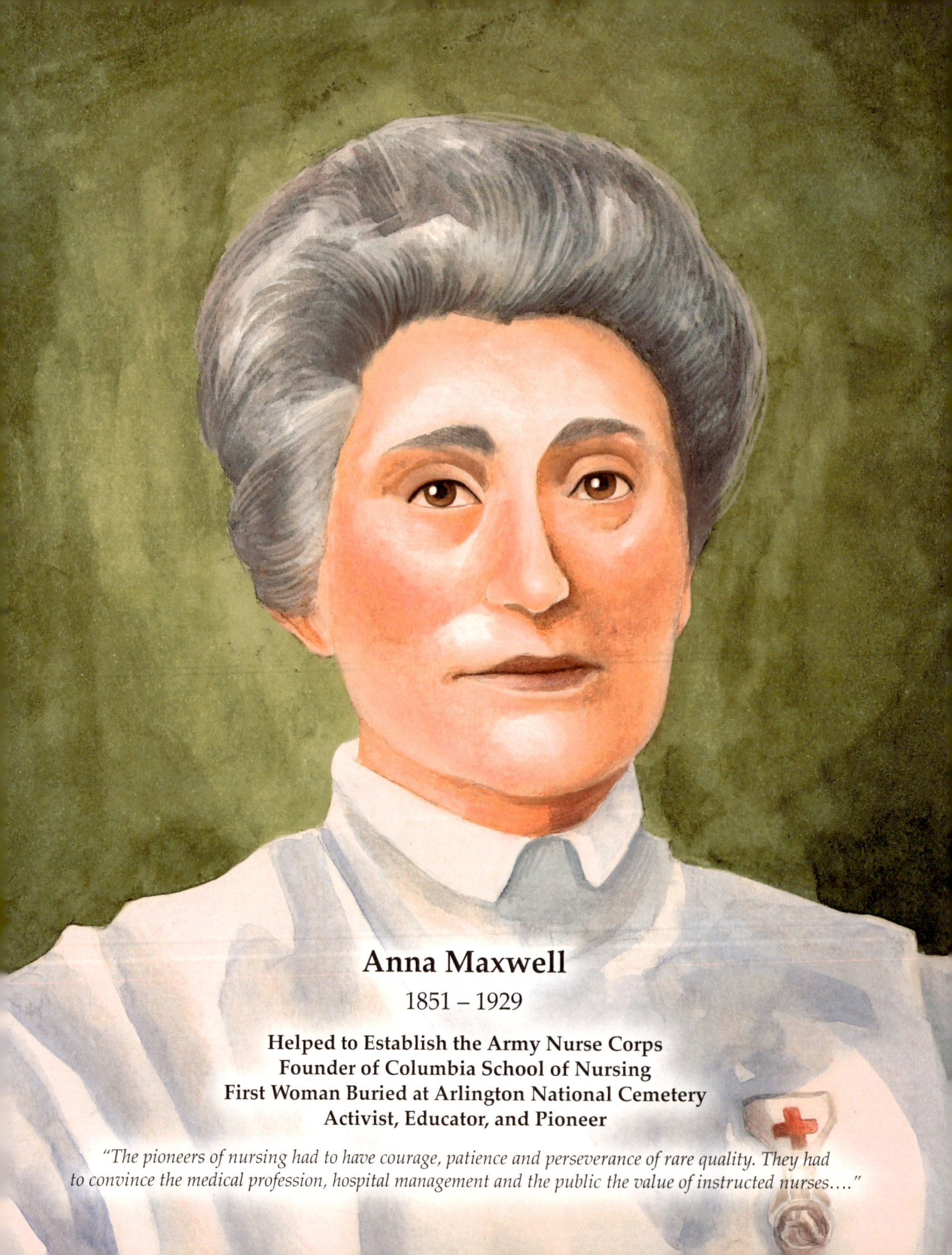

Anna Maxwell

1851 – 1929

Helped to Establish the Army Nurse Corps
Founder of Columbia School of Nursing
First Woman Buried at Arlington National Cemetery
Activist, Educator, and Pioneer

"The pioneers of nursing had to have courage, patience and perseverance of rare quality. They had to convince the medical profession, hospital management and the public the value of instructed nurses...."

Anna Caroline Maxwell was born on March 14, 1851, and was the oldest of three daughters born to Diantha Caroline Brown and John Eglington Maxwell, a Baptist minister. She was born in Bristol, New York, but spent much of her youth in King Ontario, Canada. She was tutored by her father, who had studied at the University of Edinburgh in Scotland. Anna's interest in nursing began when she took care of her ill mother.

Anna graduated from the Boston City Hospital Training School for Nurses at the age of 29 in 1880.

She moved to Canada to create a training program for nurses at Montreal General Hospital. Anna had a passion for teaching, and her exceptional organizational skills led to her having many supervisory positions. As a young nurse, she was dedicated to improving the public's opinion of the value of nurses to society. She set high standards for herself and her students. Nurse Maxwell insisted that her students come from strong family backgrounds, be well educated, and be dignified in word and appearance. She designed uniforms, capes, caps, and school pins for her students and the nurses in the Army, although she never wore a nursing cap herself. Anna is most well known for her leadership at the Presbyterian Hospital, where she directed the nursing department and school for 30 years. The school at Presbyterian Hospital would later become Columbia University School of Nursing.

During the Civil War, soldiers received nursing care from their wives, mothers, or sisters who volunteered to care for them. Clara Barton, Dorthea Dix, and Susie King Taylor were women who volunteered and whose contributions improved the conditions and survival of the soldiers, although they had no formal nurse training. Nurse Maxwell, familiar with unsanitary conditions during the Civil War, wrote to the United States Surgeon General of the Army when the Spanish American War broke out in 1898. She requested permission to bring trained nurses to care for the sick and wounded. She brought 160 nurses with her to Fort Thomas in Chickamauga, Georgia. Upon their arrival to the camp, they found soldiers living in horrible conditions. Nurse Maxwell's team of nurses cared for 1,000 ill soldiers suffering from typhoid, yellow fever, and measles. They were able to prevent the deaths of all but 67 men.

When World War I began, Nurse Maxwell was appointed to Chief Nurse of the medical unit at Presbyterian Hospital. She traveled to 3 different war zones and gathered valuable information from the hospitals she visited, which helped the United States in the medical preparations for possible war. Anna was not permitted to serve as an active duty nurse because of her age when the U.S. entered the war on April 6, 1917. Anna was 1 of 3 American nurses awarded the Médaille d'Honneur de l'Hygiène Publique, the Medal of Honor for Public Health, by the French government.

Anna knew the impact that educated and skilled nurses had on reducing suffering and preventing deaths during war. She advocated for the establishment of an Army Nurse Corps and wanted the nurses to be awarded officer rank. She also advocated for a pool of well-trained nurses to be supplied through the Red Cross in times of emergency. Congress finally approved the granting of medical rank in 1920.

Nurse Anna Caroline Maxwell never tired of promoting the profession of nursing. She shared her vision and leadership skills with the American Society of Superintendents of Training Schools for Nurses, the American Nurses Association, the International Council of Nurses, and the *American Journal of Nursing*. She is celebrated for her work in educating capable, competent, and compassionate nurses for society.

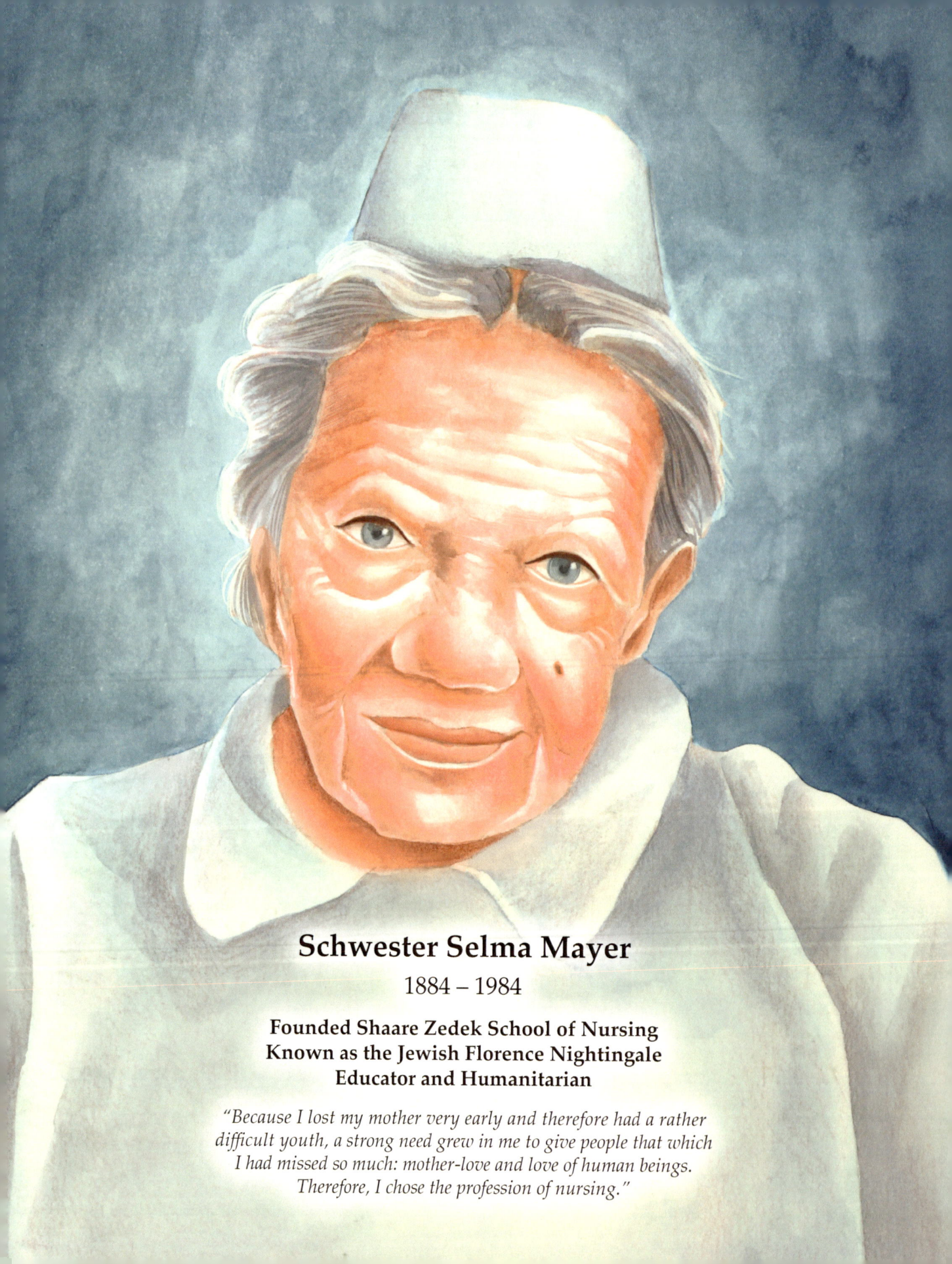

Schwester Selma Mayer

1884 – 1984

**Founded Shaare Zedek School of Nursing
Known as the Jewish Florence Nightingale
Educator and Humanitarian**

*"Because I lost my mother very early and therefore had a rather
difficult youth, a strong need grew in me to give people that which
I had missed so much: mother-love and love of human beings.
Therefore, I chose the profession of nursing."*

Selma Mayer was born on February 3, 1884, in Hanover, Germany, to a poor Jewish family. Her mother died in childbirth when Selma was 5 years old, leaving Selma and her four siblings as orphans. Selma keenly felt the loss of her mother and devoted her life to helping others.

In 1906, she began working as a nurse at Salomon Heine Hospital in Hamburg, Germany. She practiced nursing in many areas of the hospital, including pediatrics, medicine, surgery, and maternity. Seven years later, she and another nurse passed the government's nursing licensing exams. They became the first Jewish nurses to receive German State Nursing Diplomas. In Germany, a nurse is called "Schwéster," meaning "sister" in English.

During World War I, in 1916, Schwéster (sister) Selma, as she was known, was recommended to serve as a head nurse in a newly constructed hospital in Jerusalem. It was called Shaare Zedek and was the first Jewish hospital. She was 32 years old at the time, and she agreed to a 3-year contract to fulfill her war service in Palestine. It took her four weeks of traveling by train through Central Europe, Turkey, and Damascus to reach Jerusalem.

Shaare Zedek had no electricity, indoor plumbing, central heating, or gas cooking stoves. Kerosene heaters were used to warm bathwater, and paraffin lamps were used in the operating rooms. Within weeks of her arrival, Jerusalem was hit by a year-long typhoid epidemic. Typhus and meningitis were also raging in the city at the time. Additional hospital beds were needed to care for the sick, so another 110 beds were added to the 40-bed hospital to accommodate all of the patients. Desperately needing help, the hospital recruited untrained workers. Selma trained and supervised nurses and aides. She introduced German standards of nursing throughout the hospital: the wearing of white uniforms for all hospital workers, the changing of uniforms and bed sheets daily, and the daily bathing of patients. Selma worked 18-hour days and expected the same work ethic from the nursing staff.

Schwéster Selma was a tiny woman, less than 5 feet tall, yet her influence at Shaare Zedek was enormous. In addition to serving as head nurse for over 50 years, her other duties included assisting during surgeries, founding the Shaare Zedek School of Nursing and teaching all practical nursing classes, being responsible for building maintenance and ordering supplies, and overseeing the Kashrut, which were Jewish dietary laws, in the kitchen.

The original 3-year stay turned into 68 years. Selma was known for her kindness, her conscientious attention to duty, and her devotion to her patients. She often sat up all night with a critically ill patient. She never married, choosing instead to live in a sparsely furnished room in the hospital. Knowing too well the need for a mother's love, she adopted 3 girls who had been abandoned at the hospital.

In 1974, at the age of 90, the mayor of Jerusalem named Selma a "Worthy of Jerusalem." In 1975, *Time Magazine* recognized her as one of the world's "living saints" in a list that included Mother Teresa. Numerous other publications referred to her as the Jewish Florence Nightingale for her decades of selfless devotion to her patients. She has a street named in her honor in Jerusalem. She died on February 5, 1984, two days after her 100th birthday. That was the same day a special tribute had been planned to honor Salma at the hospital.

Schwéster Selma Mayer never lost the desire to give others a mother's love. Her photograph hangs in the lobby of Shaare Zedek as inspiration to follow her example.

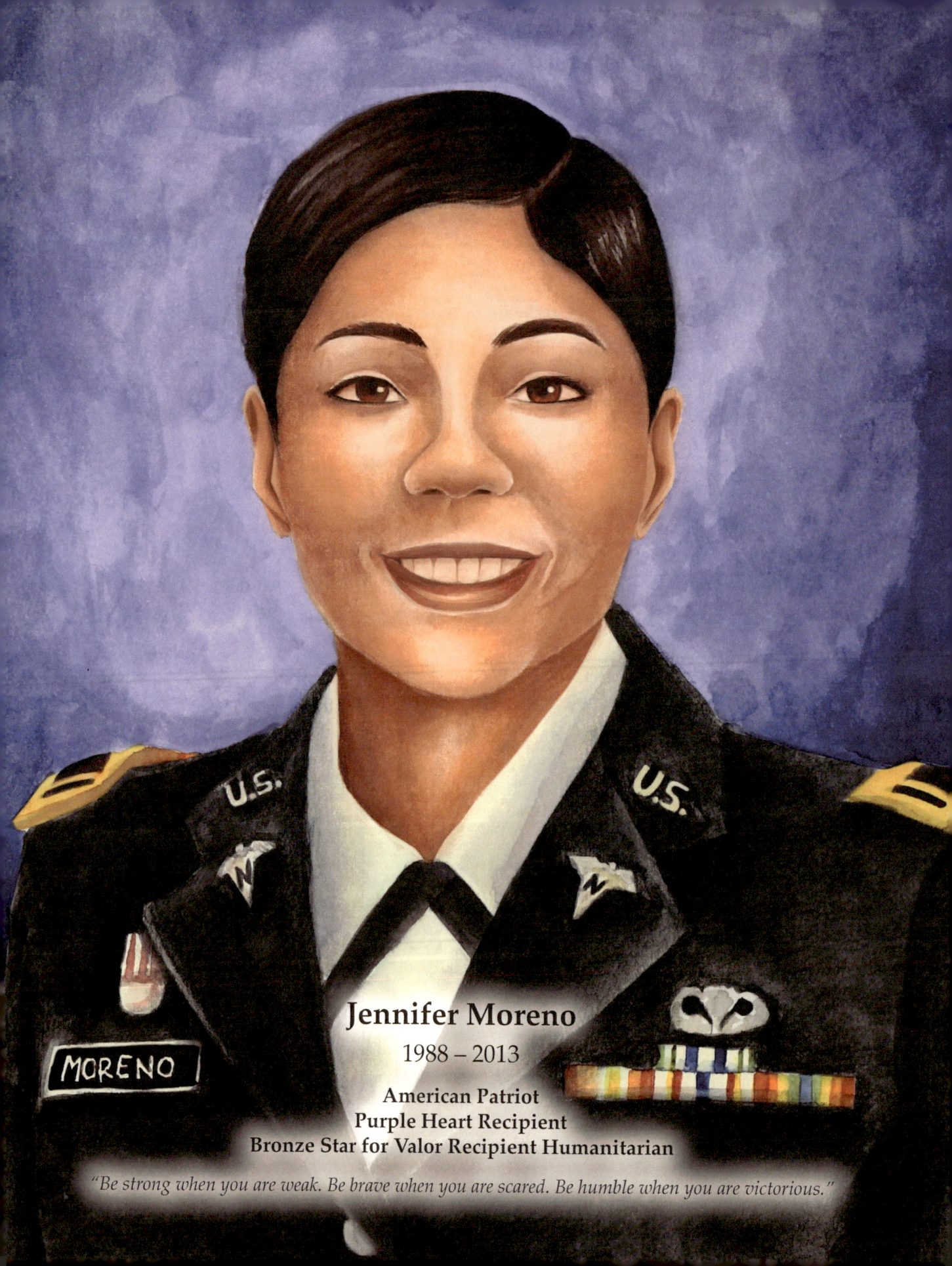

Jennifer Moreno
1988 – 2013

American Patriot
Purple Heart Recipient
Bronze Star for Valor Recipient Humanitarian

"Be strong when you are weak. Be brave when you are scared. Be humble when you are victorious."

Jennifer Moreno was born on June 25, 1988, and was one of four children born to a single immigrant mother. She graduated from San Diego High School and was the first in her family to attend college. She attended the University of San Francisco School of Nursing on a Reserve Officer Training Corps (ROTC) scholarship. She completed the Army Airborne Course at Fort Benning, Georgia, in 2009. She graduated in 2010 and was commissioned as a 1st Lieutenant in the United States Army Nurse Corps. She completed the Army Medical Officer Basic Training Course at Fort Sam Houston, Texas, and was sent to Madigan Army Base in Tacoma, Washington, to begin her career as a nurse and Army officer.

Quiet and unassuming, Jenny never wanted to bring attention to herself; instead, she wanted to showcase the accomplishments of others. She was known for her empathy, intellect, and vibrant smile. She brought a calming presence to frightened and worried patients. Her eyes conveyed confidence when a crisis was unfolding, and she skillfully organized members of the care team to save lives. She excelled at providing families with information and support, helping them understand the important activities needed to heal and recover.

First Lieutenant Moreno wanted to serve her country in a greater capacity, so she volunteered to become a member of the Cultural Support Team that would be sent to Afghanistan. The war in Afghanistan began in 2001, after the September 11th attacks that killed 3,000 people in the United States. The Taliban, a group of radical Islamists, protected Osama Bin Laden, the mastermind of the attacks. When the Taliban came to power in 1996, women lost the opportunity to travel alone or have education, employment, or healthcare. The war has been the United States' longest war, and U.S. troops have remained in Afghanistan for fear that the Taliban will provide a safe place for international terrorists to hide.

Nurse Moreno was selected from thousands of female Army officers who applied for the chance to become a member of the first-ever Female Engagement Team. Becoming a member of the multinational and multi-branch team was one of the only ways that a female soldier could participate in combat missions with the all-male Green Beret and Ranger teams. She was the first nurse ever to be selected for a mission of this type. The danger was great. One of her primary responsibilities was to interact with Afghan women and gather information that a male soldier could not get due to the cultural differences that existed in a Muslim country.

First Lieutenant Moreno had only been in Afghanistan for 3 months with the Army's 75th Ranger Regiment when a night patrol turned deadly. Jenny and 3 other soldiers were killed when a series of bombs exploded, and 30 soldiers were wounded. Nurse Moreno ran to the aid of a wounded soldier and stepped on a concealed landmine. She lived by the Soldier's Creed "I will never leave a fallen comrade." The night mission prevented a planned homicide bomber attack in the city of Kandahar, Afghanistan. Several hundreds of civilian lives were saved.

After her death, she was awarded the Bronze Star, the nation's 4th highest award for combat service, as well as the Purple Heart. She was also promoted to the rank of captain. A primary-care clinic at Fort Sam Houston, the home of Army Medicine, was renamed the Captain Jennifer M. Moreno Clinic in her memory. It is a fitting tribute to an Army nurse officer and patriot whose Army career started there.

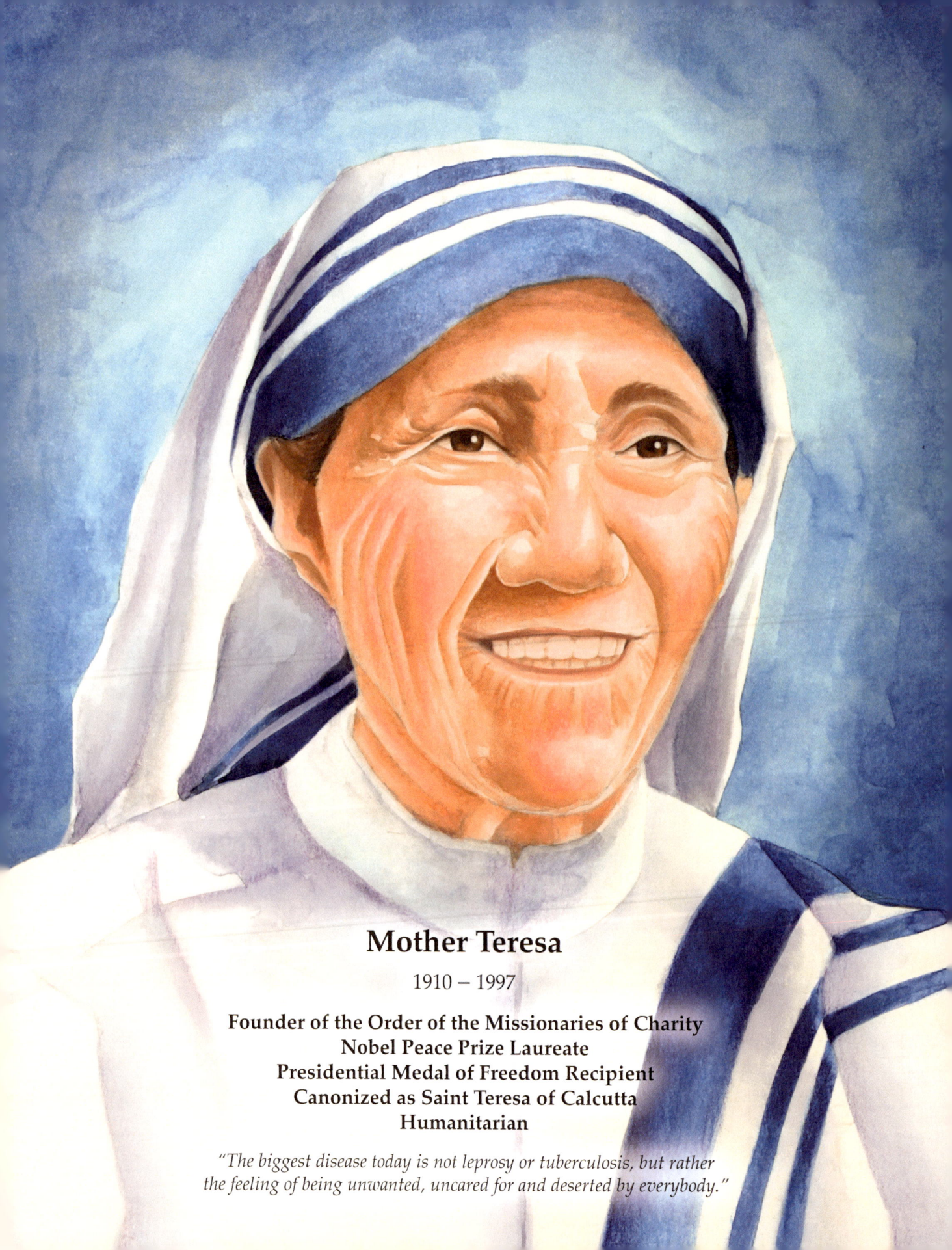

Mother Teresa

1910 – 1997

**Founder of the Order of the Missionaries of Charity
Nobel Peace Prize Laureate
Presidential Medal of Freedom Recipient
Canonized as Saint Teresa of Calcutta
Humanitarian**

"The biggest disease today is not leprosy or tuberculosis, but rather the feeling of being unwanted, uncared for and deserted by everybody."

Mother Teresa was born on August 26, 1910, in Skopje, Macedonia, and was named Anjenze (Agnes) Gonxha Bojaxhiu. Agnes was the youngest child of Nikolle and Dranafie Bojaxhi. Her mother was a homemaker; her father was a successful and influential businessman. Agnes's father died unexpectedly when she was 8, propelling her family into poverty. To provide food and housing for the family, her mother earned money by sewing and embroidering. Though the family was poor, their mother opened their home to others who were poor, hungry, and neglected. Dranafie's generosity, kindness, and compassion were lessons in love and acceptance that Agnes would share with the rest of the world.

When Agnes was 12, she felt called to become a nun, although she had never met one. She spent 6 years praying that entering religious life and serving others was her purpose. At 18, Agnes traveled to Ireland, joined the Sisters of Loreto, and then moved to India, where she dedicated her life to caring for the poorest of the poor. She chose the religious name of Teresa, after St. Therese of Lisieux, known as the patron saint of missionaries.

In Calcutta (now Kolkata), Mother Teresa's first assignment was as a teacher. Her students came from the slums, and they came to class hungry and thirsty, wearing dirty clothes. They had no food, safe drinking water, or electricity. The classroom was often a stable or an outside courtyard, and concern for her students' well-being compelled Teresa to roll up her sleeves and sweep and wash the floor before she could begin her lessons. The children watched in amazement, as cleaning was usually performed by people of the lowest status, not a nun.

Mother Teresa was dedicated to her work. Her fellow sisters became concerned about her health and encouraged her to attend a retreat in Darjeeling to rest and reflect. On the train to the retreat, Mother Teresa experienced a revelation and decided to leave the Sister of Loreto order and live among the poor. After getting approval from the Vatican, in 1948, Mother Teresa left the order and began 6 months of medical training. She never attended a formal nursing school, yet she practiced the art of nursing, caring for millions of poor and dying in India.

In 1950, she founded a new religious order: the Missionaries of Charity, whose mission was "to serve the hungry, homeless, crippled, blind, and lepers, all who feel unwanted or unloved, those who have become a burden to society, and those shunned by everyone." There is a story that has been told about a dying man who lived on the streets his entire life, and when taken to Mother Teresa's infirmary, he said, "I have lived on the streets like an animal but will die in the arms of an angel."

She was awarded the Nobel Peace Prize in 1979 for her works of mercy. She requested that the traditional banquet for the award winners be canceled, and she used the $6,000 banquet funds to host a Christmas dinner for 2,000 homeless people in India. She distributed the $190,000 award to the homeless in her adopted country of India. President Reagan bestowed the Presidential Medal of Freedom on Mother Teresa, and on September 4, 2016, Pope Francis proclaimed Mother Theresa a saint.

Mother Teresa is one of the most beloved and admired humanitarians of the 20th century. She believed that each person was worthy of love, compassion, and respect. The United Nations General Assembly declared September 5, the anniversary of her death, as International Day of Charity to promote acts of kindness and generosity throughout the world.

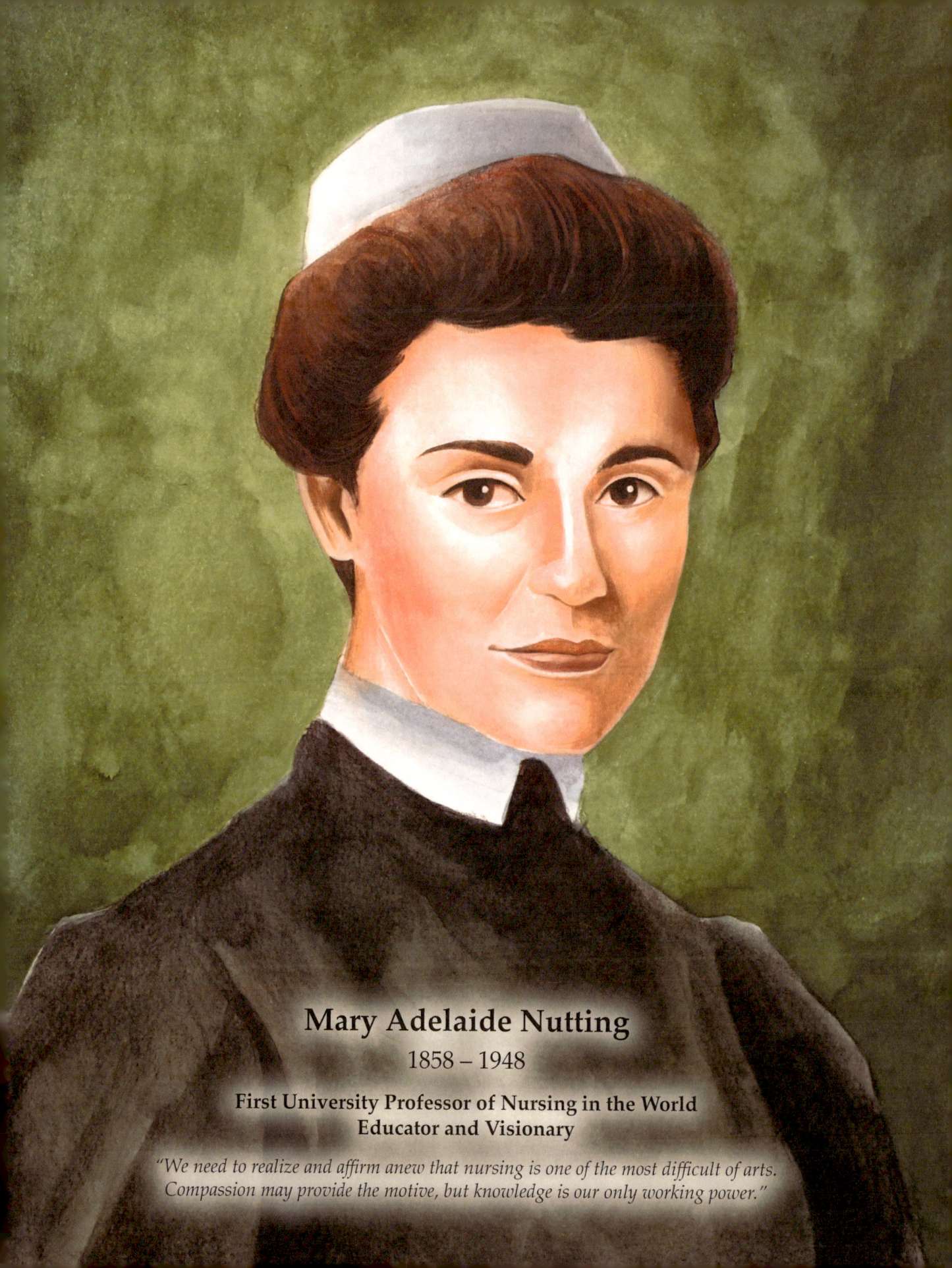

Mary Adelaide Nutting

1858 – 1948

**First University Professor of Nursing in the World
Educator and Visionary**

*"We need to realize and affirm anew that nursing is one of the most difficult of arts.
Compassion may provide the motive, but knowledge is our only working power."*

Mary Adelaide Nutting was born on November 1, 1858, in Waterloo, Canada. She was the fourth of five children born to Harriet Sophia Peasley and Vespasian Nutting. Her father was a warm and loving man but struggled to provide for his family as a county clerk. Adelaide's mother was a seamstress and used her talent to help support the family. Her mother wanted her children to be well educated in the music and arts and to be challenged academically. Adelaide attended a local academy and a convent school even though money was tight. She attended a boarding school in Quebec, where she became an accomplished pianist and singer. She taught music for a year at an all girl's school in Newfoundland where Armin, her sister, was principal.

Adelaide spent much of her young adulthood living at home, helping her family with their finances. She had big dreams for her life, as she had watched her smart and gifted mother keep her thoughts and opinions about the world to herself. While women in the 1850s could work outside the home, they could not vote, have a bank account, or own property. In 1884, Harriet became ill, and Adelaide took care of her. She often felt inadequate, as she believed there was more she could be doing for her mother if she only had the proper training.

She read in the newspaper about a training school for nurses that was opening in the United States. Based on Florence Nightingale's principles, it would provide lodging and a small wage while studying. Adelaide was 1 of 17 women to make up the first class at the Johns Hopkins Hospital Training School for Nurses in Baltimore, Maryland. She entered the program the day before her 31st birthday.

Adelaide was ambitious and decided she would not marry or have children. She wanted to have a career that would allow her to be independent, and she believed nursing would provide that type of life. She graduated in 1891 and began working as head nurse with the famed Doctor William Osler, one of the founders of Johns Hopkins Hospital, who was considered the "Father of Modern Medicine." Adelaide was the first nurse to be registered in the state of Maryland.

Nurse Nutting spent half of her professional career at Johns Hopkins, becoming assistant superintendent of nurses and then becoming superintendent and director of the nursing school. Adelaide improved nursing education by introducing an 8-hour day, a 3-year course of study, and a well-prepared faculty. She also created a 6-month pre-nursing class in which the students learned and practiced skills before caring for patients in the hospital. She established scholarships for low income students, encouraged students to learn about public health nursing, and created a nursing library at Johns Hopkins. This led to her writing a multi-volume book with Lavina L. Dock titled *The History of Nursing*. Adelaide believed that nurses needed to be reading professional literature and was one of the founders of the *American Journal of Nursing*.

In 1907, Adelaide became a full-time professor of institutional management at Teachers College, Columbia University. This title was later changed to Professor of Nursing Education. Under her leadership, Columbia University prepared thousands of women by giving them new concepts for caring for the sick, helping them understand their professional and civic responsibilities in keeping the nation healthy.

During World War I, Adelaide responded to President Woodrow Wilson's request for assistance and chaired a committee to make sure that both civilians and soldiers had necessary supplies.

Nurse Mary Adelaide Nutting is widely thought to be one of the most influential nurses of all time.

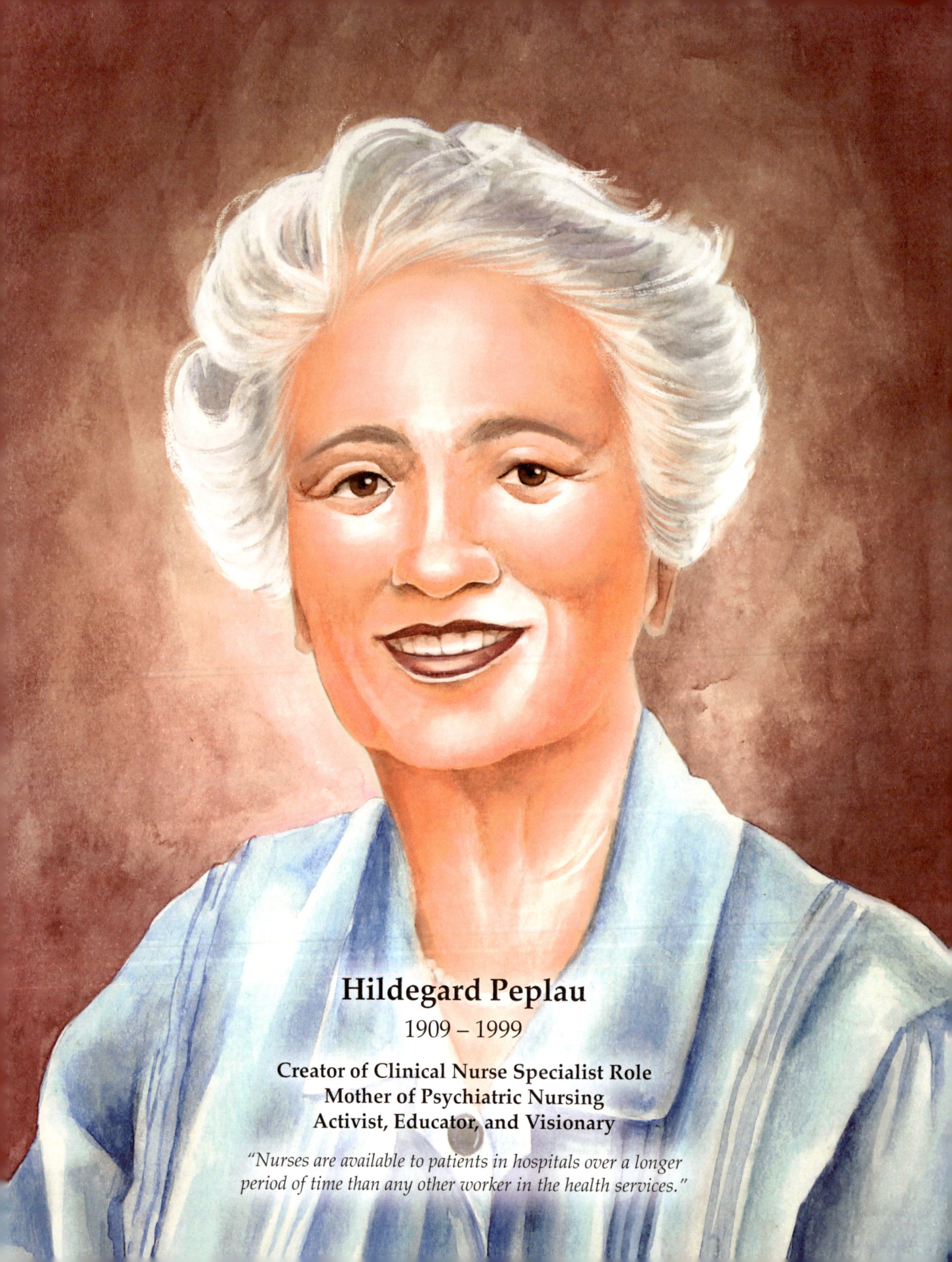

Hildegard Peplau

1909 – 1999

Creator of Clinical Nurse Specialist Role
Mother of Psychiatric Nursing
Activist, Educator, and Visionary

"Nurses are available to patients in hospitals over a longer
period of time than any other worker in the health services."

Hildegarde Elisabeth Peplau was born in Reading, Pennsylvania, on September 1, 1909, to immigrant parents. Her parents were both from Poland but did not meet until they came to the United States. Her father was a firefighter, and her mother was a homemaker. Her mother worked hard to help with the family finances by selling baked goods, working in a shirt factory, and cleaning other people's homes. Her parents had a strong work ethic and were proud that they could provide for their six children. Hilda, as she liked to be called, lived through the 1918 Spanish Flu epidemic that infected more than 500 million people in the world. This experience had a great impact on Hilda, as she witnessed the suffering and death of her neighbors.

In 1920, the 19th Amendment, which gave women the right to vote, was passed. While this was an important step in the advancement of women, there were still few career opportunities available to women. Women could marry, enter the convent, or become teachers, secretaries, or nurses. Hilda chose to become a nurse. She graduated from the Pottstown Hospital School of Nursing in 1931.

She began her nursing career working as a bedside nurse in hospitals in Pennsylvania and New York City. She also worked as a nurse at a summer camp in New York, which led to her next position as a school nurse at Bennington College in Vermont. She was promoted to Head Nurse of the College Health Service because of her leadership skills and the excellent care she provided. She graduated from Bennington College with a bachelor's degree in interpersonal psychology in 1943. She had the opportunity to study with many famous psychiatrists who taught her about the importance of forming relationships with patients in order to help them heal and recover from illnesses.

Hilda joined the Army Nurse Corps in 1943 because she believed she needed to serve her country during World War II. She was sent to England and worked along English and American psychiatrists who were learning much about mental health. Many years later, she would work with these men again to improve the mental healthcare system in the United States, which led to the passage of the National Mental Health Act of 1946.

Nurse Peplau continued her studies and earned a master's degree in psychiatric nursing and a doctorate in education from Teachers College, Columbia University. She also completed studies to become certified as a psychoanalyst, helping people deal with memories that affected their emotional well-being. Hilda designed a class for graduate nursing students who had an interest in psychiatric nursing. She also wrote a book about her opinions on how nurses can best develop relationships with their patients. Hildegard had to wait for four years to find a company who would publish her book, as she did not have a doctor as a co-author.

The field of psychiatric nursing was influenced by Nurse Peplau's thinking, teaching, and writings. She taught nurses to think of themselves as compassionate strangers entering people's lives when they are frightened, worried, and sick, and she helped nurses use their knowledge about relationships to help them get better.

Many scholars in nursing believe that Hildegard Peplau's life and work brought about the greatest changes in nursing practice since Florence Nightingale.

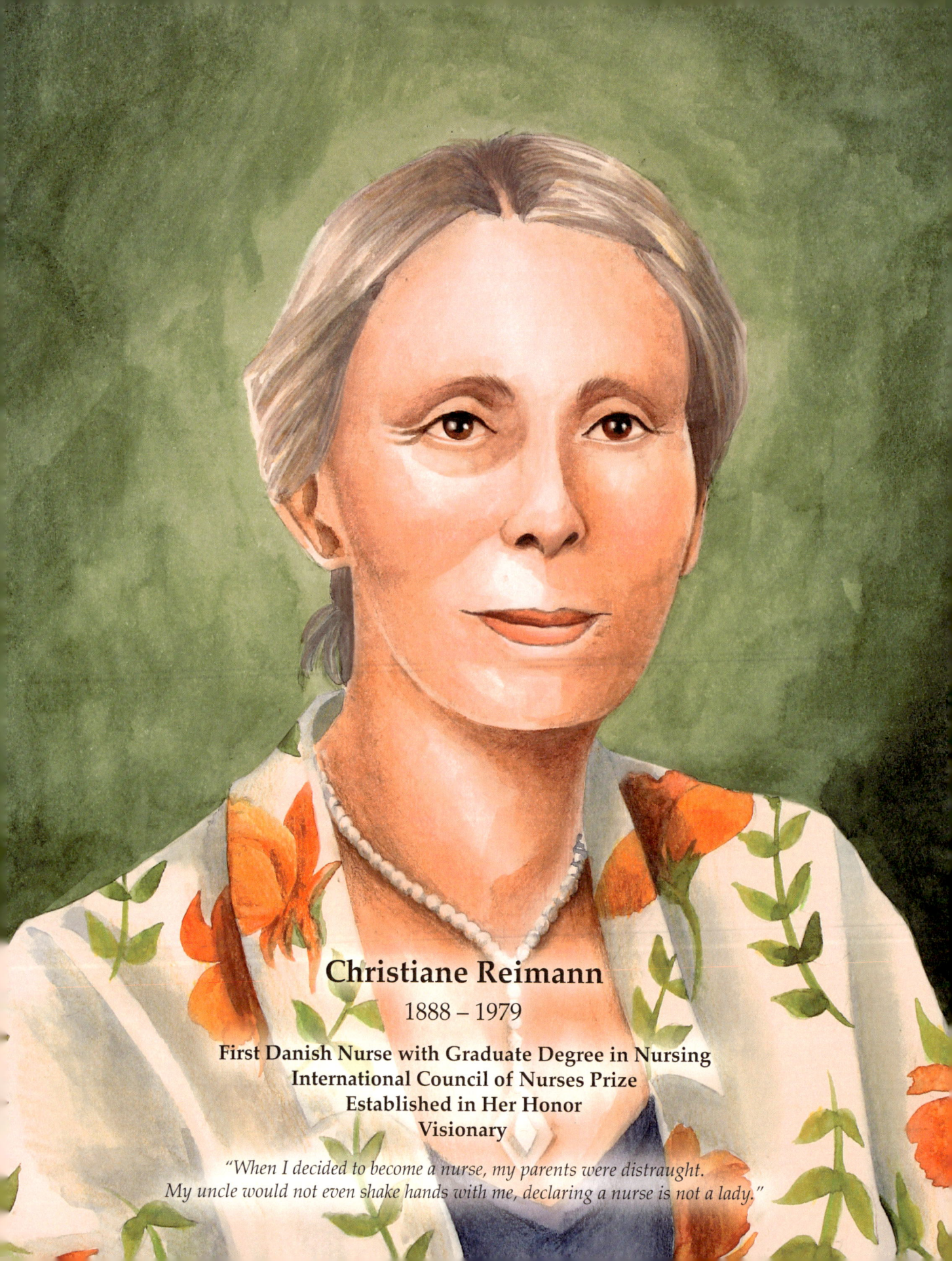

Christiane Reimann

1888 – 1979

First Danish Nurse with Graduate Degree in Nursing
International Council of Nurses Prize
Established in Her Honor
Visionary

"When I decided to become a nurse, my parents were distraught.
My uncle would not even shake hands with me, declaring a nurse is not a lady."

Christiane Christian Reimann was born in Copenhagen, Denmark, on May 6, 1888, the daughter of wealthy parents. Her father, Carl Christian Reimann, was a stockbroker, and her mother, Margit Meisterlin Reimann, managed the household. Her upbringing kept with the upper-class norms of the time. The expected path for an upper-class daughter was to prepare to become a wife and mother.

Christiane completed her basic schooling at age 16. The next nine years were spent at home, taking lessons in singing, piano playing, and music theory, with the exception of two years in Germany and England to learn the languages.

When she was 25, Christiane announced that she would become a nurse, a decision her family strongly opposed. Becoming a nurse was only acceptable if the woman had no prospects for marriage. Christiane's mind was made up, though, and no amount of disapproval from her family could change her mind.

Christiane graduated in 1916 from Bispebjerg Hospital Nursing School and sailed on the first postwar ship from Copenhagen to New York in order to pursue a higher education in nursing. By 1925, she had obtained both a bachelor's and master's degree in nursing from Teachers College, Columbia University. Thus, she was the first ever graduate-prepared Danish nurse.

Despite the great differences in nursing around the world, Christiane believed nurses in every country should be connected. The International Council of Nursing (ICN) was founded in 1899 and was the first international organization for healthcare professionals. Christiane originally joined ICN as a volunteer secretary, but later she became its first paid officer. This new position suited her. She used her fluency in other languages, her intelligence, and her great wealth to make ICN a true international voice for nursing. She established strong relationships with governmental and public health organizations and the Red Cross. She used her own money to travel extensively so she could partner with national nursing organizations. Through her leadership, ICN expanded from 13 to 29 national organization participants.

Seeing the need for an international nursing journal, Nurse Reimann founded one, funding it and writing most of its articles. To support the journal, now called the *International Nursing Review*, she created, at her own cost, a library at ICN headquarters that lent books internationally. These efforts, usually acted upon without consulting the other members of the ICN board of directors, were a constant source of irritation to her colleagues. In 1934, pleading poor health, she left her position. She moved to Italy and married a German psychiatrist. The marriage ended in divorce. Christiane spent the rest of her life in Syracuse, Italy, tending a citrus farm.

Christiane continued to follow the ICN events. In 1967, she offered the organization her villa as a retreat, but necessary repairs would have been too expensive to maintain. She then offered ICN part of her fortune to establish a prestigious international prize. True to form, her headstrong and uncompromising personality forced the negotiations to drag out for over a decade.

The first Christiane Reimann Prize was awarded in 1979, 6 years after her death. The prize is awarded every 4 years to one or more nurses who have made a significant impact on the nursing profession internationally or through the nursing profession for the benefit of humanity. The prize, a substantial cash award and a hand-painted statue of a nurse, is known all over the world as one of nursing's most prestigious awards.

The unwavering, headstrong heiress believed in the tremendous potential of nursing and ICN. That, in itself, is the great prize.

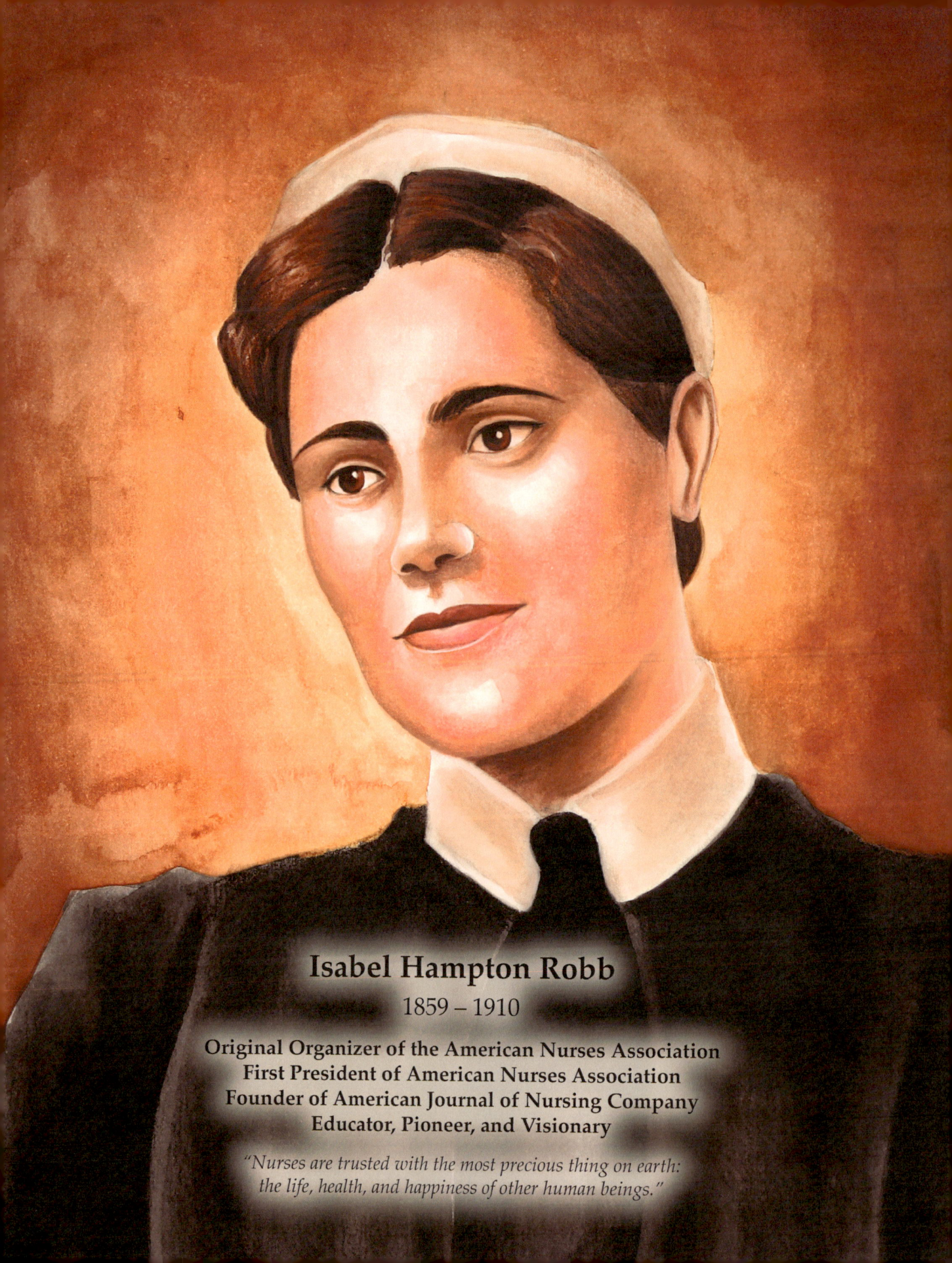

Isabel Hampton Robb

1859 – 1910

Original Organizer of the American Nurses Association
First President of American Nurses Association
Founder of American Journal of Nursing Company
Educator, Pioneer, and Visionary

*"Nurses are trusted with the most precious thing on earth:
the life, health, and happiness of other human beings."*

Isabel Adams Hampton was born in Welland, Ontario, on August 26, 1859. She was the fourth of seven children born to Samuel James and Sarah Mary Lay Hampton. Her parents were originally from Cornwall, England. At 17, Isabel became a teacher in rural Ontario, where she taught for 3 years. Isabel developed a reputation for setting high standards. She had a presence in the classroom that made even the most disobedient students behave. While teaching, Isabel continued her own education, receiving instruction in the liberal arts and mathematics by the headmaster of the Collegiate Institute at St. Catherine's in Ontario. After her teaching contract ended, Isabel applied to the Bellevue Hospital Training School for Nurses in New York City.

While a student at Bellevue, Isabel wanted to learn as much as she could. She was constantly studying her notes, reading books, and asking questions of the doctors while at the hospital. Isabel wanted to be the best nurse possible, and she knew that she needed to have a good understanding of how the body worked and what nursing care was needed for the patient to get better.

Upon graduation from Bellevue in 1883, Isabel filled in for the superintendent of nurses at the Women's Hospital in New York. Isabel traveled to Rome to work for 2 years at St. Paul's House in Rome, a place where English and American travelers could receive care. She returned to the US and worked as a private-duty nurse to a wealthy family in New Jersey. In 1886, she moved to Chicago to become superintendent of the Illinois Training School for Nurses at Cook County Hospital, and she began her work that would change the way nurses were educated in this country. She required that students receive grades, and she arranged clinical experiences at other hospitals aside from their training hospital. In 1889, she was recruited to Baltimore to become the first Superintendent of the Johns Hopkins Training School for Nurses, which was just opening.

Nurse Hampton created a nursing program that prepared excellent nurses and taught them how to be leaders and challenge current thinking. She standardized the nursing curriculum requiring 3 years of study. She established 8-hour workdays, reduced the number of hours in the wards from 56 hours per week to 40, and started a nurses' journal club. She published her first book, which described exactly what students needed to learn. Her textbook, called *Nursing: Its Principles and Practices*, was the first of its kind ever published and included chapters on proper hygiene in hospitals, medical emergencies, and infectious diseases. These topics are still taught today.

In June of 1894, Isabel left Johns Hopkins to marry Dr. Hunter Robb, who was the newly appointed professor of gynecology at Case Western Reserve University. They were married in London, and Isabel carried a bouquet of flowers sent to her by Florence Nightingale.

Many nurse leaders feared that Isabel's contributions to nursing would come to an end, as she began devoting her time to raising her two sons, Hampton and Phillip. This was not the case, though, as Isabel became a member of the Board of Lady Managers of Lakeside Hospital in Cleveland, which later became Frances Payne Bolton School of Nursing, Case Western Reserve University. Isabel provided lectures at the hospital school and continued her writing and professional organization work. Her leadership helped create the International Council of Nurses, and she served as the first president of the American Nurses Association.

Nurse Isabel Hampton Robb's genius allowed her to see the possibilities for the profession of nursing decades before others. She is considered one of the greatest nursing educators of all time.

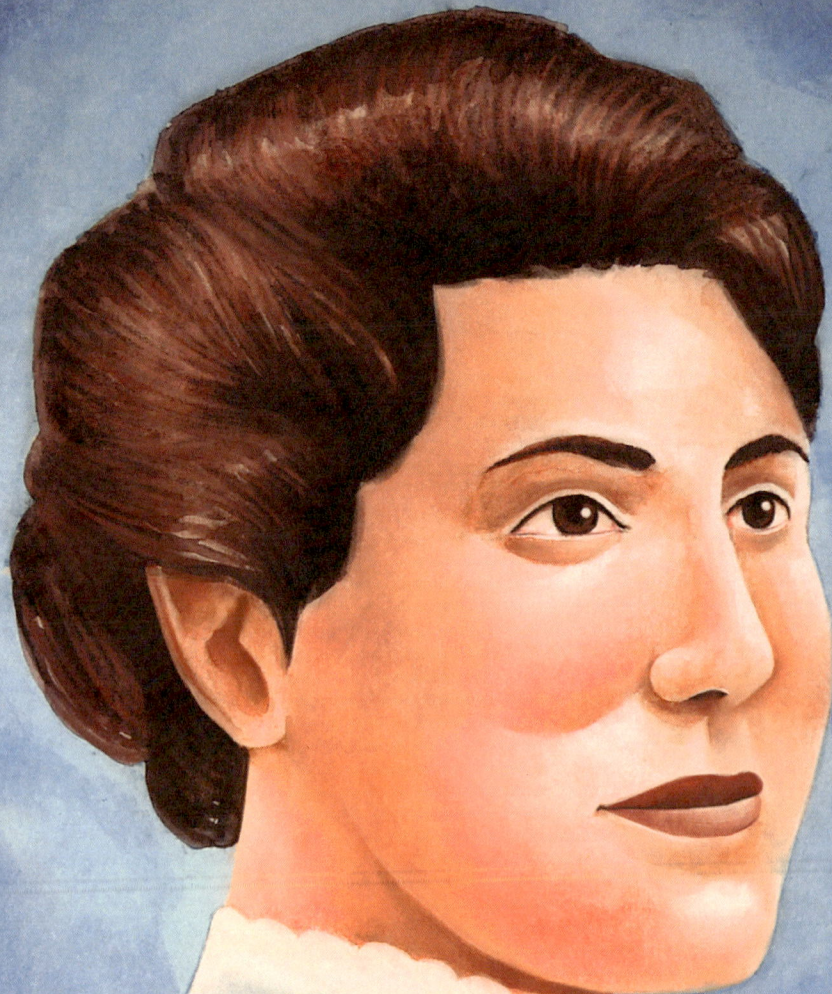

Lina Rogers

1870 – 1946

First School Nurse
Activist, Author, and Educator

"A sensible school nurse, with good judgment, discretion and enthusiasm,
may be a powerful factor in the general improvement of a community."

Lina Lavanche Rogers was born in Ontario, Canada, in 1870. Little is known about her early child-hood. In 1896, Lina graduated from the School of Nursing of the Hospital for Sick Children in Toronto, Canada. She continued her education at the Royal Victoria Hospital in Montreal. She left Canada and moved to Atlanta, Georgia, to become the Superintendent of Nurses at Grady Hospital. Lina became aware of the work of Nurse Lillian Wald, a crusader for public health, and moved to New York City to live and work at the Henry Street Settlement.

Between 1870 and 1900, approximately 12 million immigrants came to the United States. New York City experienced such a rapid growth in population that many poor parts of the city became overcrowded, which led to unsanitary conditions and widespread disease. New York required that all school-age children attend school. Many of the children living in such poor conditions brought infections to school that were highly contagious. They unknowingly infected their class-mates, which resulted in empty classrooms. On any given day, thousands of children would not be in school.

Two influential public officials sought advice from Nurse Lillian Wald and the other nurses at Henry Street Settlement, asking for ways to improve the screening of children when they came to school. Nurse Wald recommended that a nurse be placed in the schools to treat the children. The nurse could provide follow-up care by visiting the children in their homes. The visit would allow the nurse to observe the home, check on other members living there, and provide an opportunity to teach the parents. Nurse Wald negotiated and created a permanent school nurse position that would be paid for by public funds if the 30-day trial run she proposed was successful. Lina Rogers was selected as the first school nurse.

Nurse Rogers began attending to the health of 100,000 students in four schools in October of 1902. During the 30-day trial, Lina made an impact. She was able to examine and treat children, and they were able to return to school. After school, Lina would visit the children's homes and teach their parents about hand washing, hygiene, and eliminating waste products. At the end of October, Lina was awarded the New York City Board of Education's first school nurse position. The school nurse program grew rapidly, and by 1914, there was a nurse working in every school.

While screening and treating children at school and visiting their homes, Lina was often heart-broken by what she witnessed. She soon realized that the children were missing school for reasons other than illness. Many were absent because they did not have shoes or food, or they were working in horrific conditions. Lina worked with social services to help them get food, clothing, and safe employment.

Nurse Rogers continued to influence the health and lives of the school children of New York City. She lobbied for health education and taught teachers how to teach their students about hygiene, nutrition, and growth and development. She introduced the use of paper towels for hand drying to prevent the spread of disease. She was the first to emphasize dental health and hearing testing in schools. She developed many protocols that were used to establish regulations for school nursing.

Lina returned to Canada in 1913 to begin a nursing program that included doctors, dentists, and nurses. The focus of the curriculum was comprehensive school health services. She married Dr. William E. Struthers and retired from the practice of school nursing. She continued to share her knowledge during retirement by writing the first textbook for school nurses.

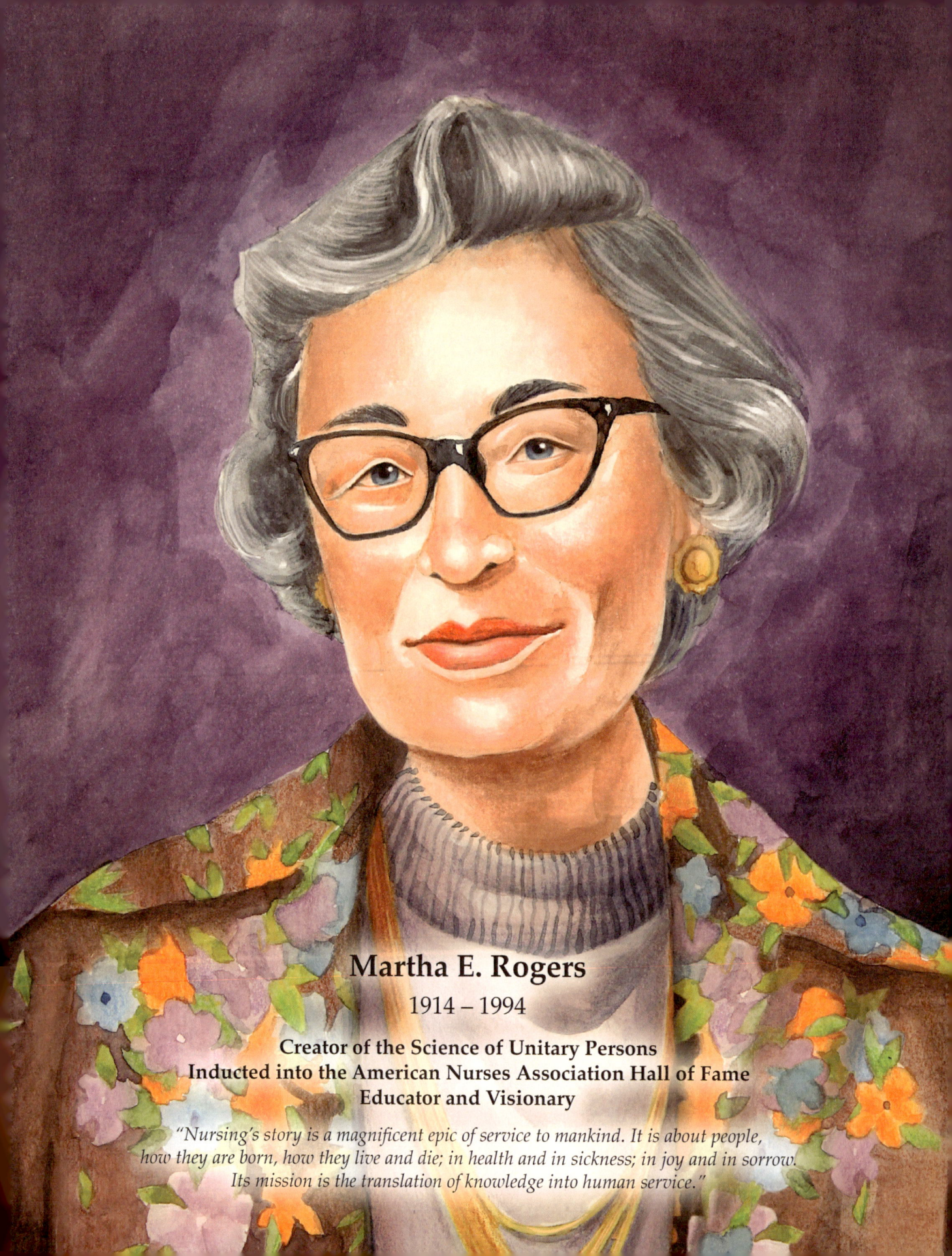

Martha E. Rogers

1914 – 1994

**Creator of the Science of Unitary Persons
Inducted into the American Nurses Association Hall of Fame
Educator and Visionary**

*"Nursing's story is a magnificent epic of service to mankind. It is about people,
how they are born, how they live and die; in health and in sickness; in joy and in sorrow.
Its mission is the translation of knowledge into human service."*

Martha Elizabeth Rogers was born on May 12, 1914, in Dallas, Texas. She shares the May 12th birthdate with Florence Nightingale. She was the oldest of four children. Many of her admirers consider her the 20th-century Nightingale because of her tireless work to place nursing in a positive position within healthcare.

Martha had a passion and thirst for knowledge at an early age. She knew the Greek alphabet by age 10. By 6th grade, she had read all 20 volumes of *The Child's Book of Knowledge*, and then she started with the 32 *Encyclopedia Britannica* books, which contained all of the facts known in 1926. She read about various topics, including anthropology, archaeology, cosmology, ethnography, astronomy, ethics, psychology, philosophy, and aesthetics. During her senior year in high school, she took a college-level algebra course and was the only woman in the class.

Martha studied medicine for two years at the University of Tennessee, Knoxville, before transferring into nursing. She was interested in addressing social welfare issues. She received a diploma from the Knoxville General Hospital School of Nursing in 1936, and she got a Public Health Nursing degree from George Peabody College in 1937. In 1945, she sold her car to pay for tuition so she could obtain her master's degree from Teachers College, Columbia University. She worked as a public health nurse in Michigan, Connecticut, New York, and Arizona prior to her doctoral studies. She received a master's in public health and then a doctorate from Johns Hopkins University in 1954, and then she was recruited to head the New York University (NYU) nursing program.

As NYU's head of nursing for 21 years, Rogers carved a role for science development within nursing. She created the first PhD program in nursing and recruited many graduate students in order to advance her ideas. Based on her knowledge of science and humanities, she developed a unique model of nursing called "The Science of Unitary Persons." She introduced new concepts within nursing—ideas that nurses had never previously considered. She wanted nurses to understand that a person's health was influenced by his environment. She introduced nurses to concepts with big words and new ideas. She wanted nurses to consider open systems, wholeness, transcendence, human environmental energy fields, rhythms, synchrony, pan-dimensionality, and synergy. Rogers described nursing as the study of unitary, irreducible, indivisible, human and environmental fields. She believed that nursing existed to serve people and assist them in achieving their very best health.

Martha Rogers, as a person, was often considered just as radical as her nursing science ideas. She nearly always wore purple because purple wavelengths were the most complex on the light spectrum. She often donned a white mink coat, even on treks to the state offices to lobby for radical changes in legislation to advance nursing. She believed in herself and exuded a confidence in her own ideas and knowledge that was admired worldwide. Many referred to her as a genius. She imagined nurses in space and wrote about space-based nursing before others even thought of going to space.

She was an accomplished writer and speaker, authoring several books and articles and speaking around the world, sharing her strong beliefs about nursing. She never compromised her beliefs in the value of nursing to the public. Her strong public health background led her to advocate for nurses serving in the communities in which they lived rather than assuming traditional hospital roles.

Nurse Martha Rogers received several accolades throughout her career, including several honorary doctorates. She was inducted into the American Nurses Association Hall of Fame 2 years after her death in 1996.

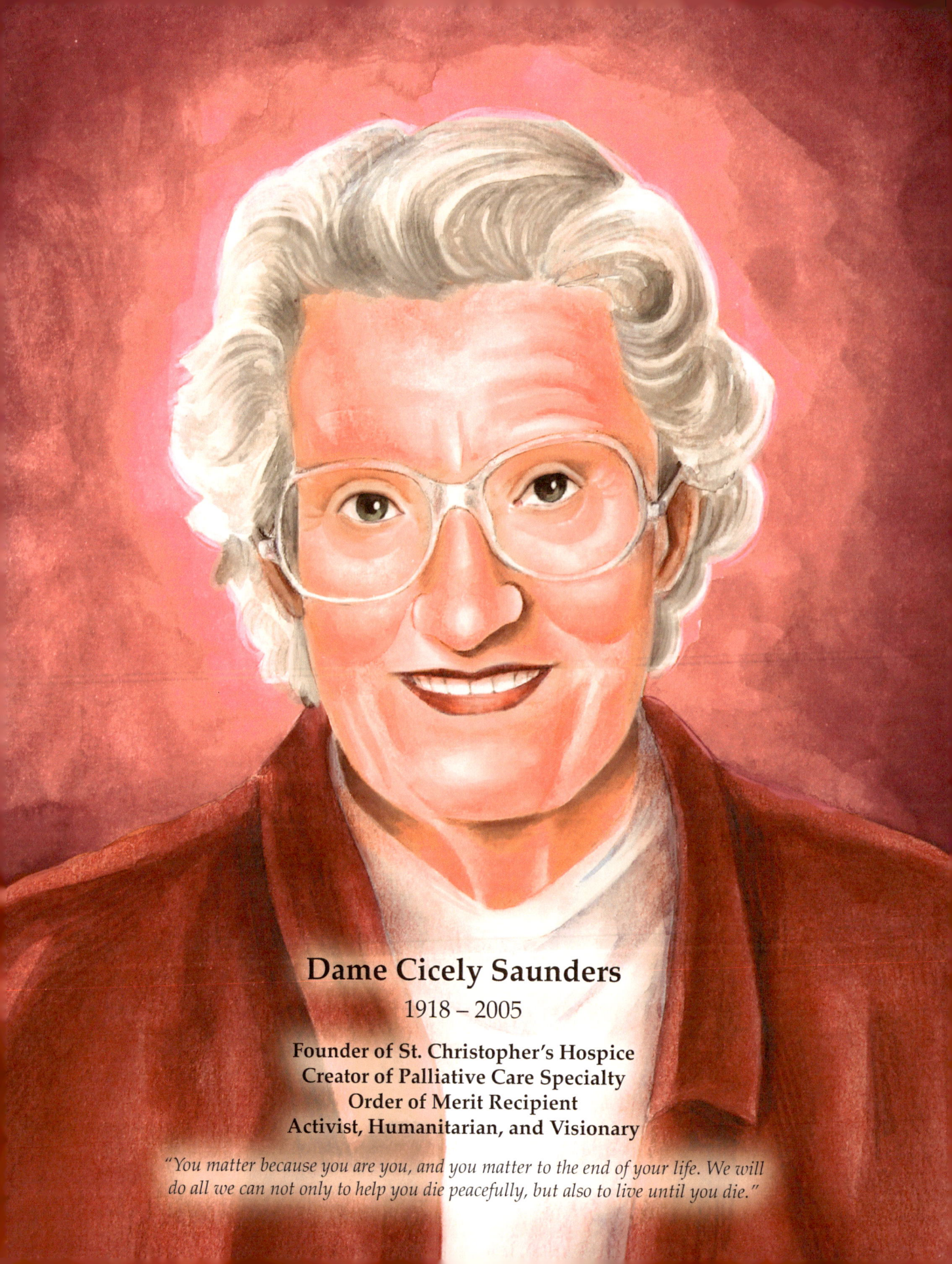

Dame Cicely Saunders

1918 – 2005

**Founder of St. Christopher's Hospice
Creator of Palliative Care Specialty
Order of Merit Recipient
Activist, Humanitarian, and Visionary**

"You matter because you are you, and you matter to the end of your life. We will do all we can not only to help you die peacefully, but also to live until you die."

Cicely Mary Strode Saunders was born in England on June 22, 1918, to Mary Christian Knight and Philip Gordon Saunders. She was the oldest of three children and was her parents' only daughter. As a child, she was taller than other girls her age and always felt left out because of her height. This experience allowed her to appreciate the suffering of those who never felt like they fit in. Cicely studied politics, philosophy, and economics at St. Anne's College, the women's college at Oxford. Cicely stopped her studies when England entered World War II. She decided to become a nurse to help her country and care for the wounded soldiers. She worked and studied at Nightingale School of Nursing for four years.

After the war, Cicely returned to St. Anne's College, completed her studies, and received certification as a medical social worker in 1947. While working as a social worker, Cicely met and fell in love with a patient who had escaped from the Warsaw Ghetto, an area in Poland where German Nazis had forced all Jewish people to live. He was dying of cancer and left Cicely a sizeable amount of money. The money and relationship provided her with the opportunity to improve the care of the dying.

As a social worker, Cicely moved to London and experienced death, loss, and grief. She experienced the death of her father and other patients and friends. This put her in a state of "pathological grieving" but also helped her realize that she wanted to start a hospice that served cancer patients. Unfortunately, she was told that her ideas of medicine and pain control for ill and dying people would not be accepted unless she was a doctor, so Cicely, having been a nurse and a social worker, became a doctor in 1957. As a doctor, she worked with patients who were terminally ill but still felt she was not doing enough.

In 1967, 11 years after thinking about the project and finding the financing to open it, St. Christopher's Hospice was opened. Hospice care is provided to patients who have a terminal, or life-ending, illness. It is intended to help ease the pain as people transition to dying. This was important to Cicely; her experiences with death had shown her that "as the body becomes weaker, so the spirit becomes stronger."

St. Christopher's House was a research and teaching hospice whose caregivers emphasized pain and symptom control, compassionate care, and teaching and research, and it pioneered the specialty of nursing and medicine called "palliative care." The philosophy at St. Christopher's House was that "you matter because you are you and you matter until the last moment of your life."

Cicely's vision was revolutionary, her dedication to her dream steadfast. She was recognized for her work and granted damehood, a title of honor bestowed by Queen Elizabeth, in 1979. Ten years later, she was appointed to the Order of Merit, a recognition given to the members of the Commonwealth for distinguished service in the arts, literature, sciences, and armed forces. In 2001, she was awarded the Conrad. N. Hilton Humanitarian Prize, the world's largest humanitarian award. She also found love at the age of 61, marrying Marian Bohusz-Szyszko, a Polish professor and artist.

Dame Cicely Saunders used her knowledge and experiences of feeling alone, grieving, and suffering to change the way dying patients are ushered into death. Her work is carried on by the thousands of nurses, doctors, and social workers she taught, who had the good fortune to learn from her.

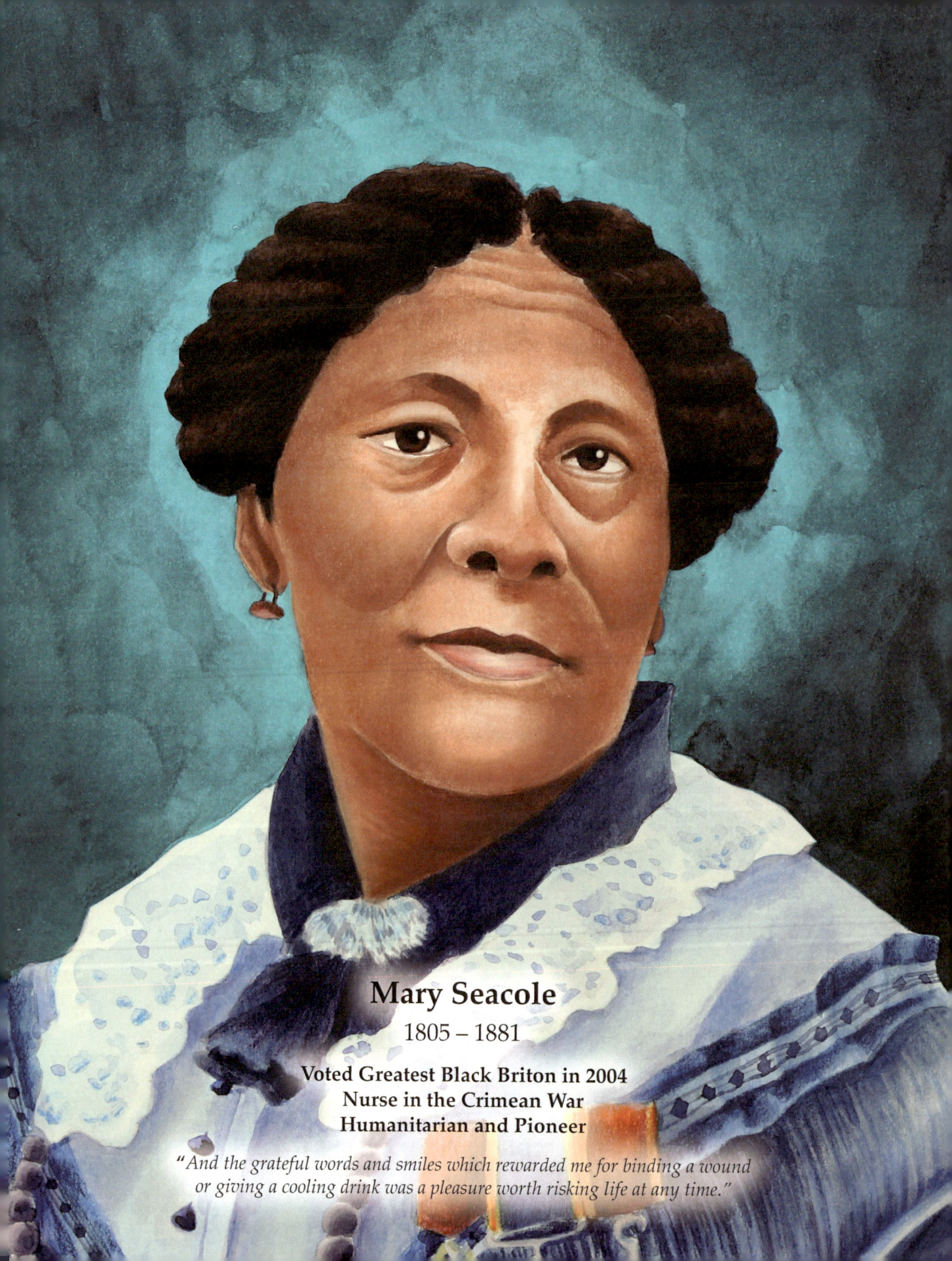

Mary Seacole

1805 – 1881

Voted Greatest Black Briton in 2004
Nurse in the Crimean War
Humanitarian and Pioneer

"And the grateful words and smiles which rewarded me for binding a wound
or giving a cooling drink was a pleasure worth risking life at any time."

Mary Jane Grant was born in Kingston, Jamaica. Her mother was Jamaican, and her father was Scottish. Mary's father was a soldier, and her mother set up a boarding house in her village. In the early 1800s, boarding houses were places where people could rent a room for a few nights or several months. Mary spent her childhood observing her mother taking care of sick and wounded soldiers who often stayed at the boarding house. After hearing stories from her father's time as a soldier, Mary dreamed of making a difference in times of war and found herself thinking a lot about those who suffered during wartime.

There were no schools for Mary to attend to learn to become a nurse. Instead, she learned by watching her mother work. When Mary was about 12 years old, she started helping her mother take care of the people who rented rooms at the boarding house, and she began to learn what it takes to be a nurse. She admired her mother, who was able to calm people who were afraid, comfort those who were thirsty or in pain, and bandage wounds to prevent infections.

In 1836, Mary married Edwin Horatio Hamilton Seacole. They opened a store in Black River, a small Jamaican village, and after eight years of marriage, Edwin became extremely ill. Mary took care of him, but even with the best nursing care, Edwin did not survive. After her husband's death, Mary took over her mother's boarding house. Soldiers often stayed at her boarding house to recover from infectious diseases such as cholera and yellow fever, and Mary's reputation as a skillful nurse and healer grew.

The Crimean War broke out in Europe in 1853, when Russia invaded Turkey. Mary was living in London during this time. She felt an overwhelming calling to travel to the war zone, so she volunteered to help care for the soldiers. However, her request was denied by the War Office. After several rejections to join Florence Nightingale's group of nurses, Mary, at the age of 49, used her own money and asked for donations from friends to fund her passage to Crimea. She opened the "British Hotel" close to the front lines. There, soldiers were offered nutritious food, given an opportunity to recuperate in comfortable surroundings, and received herbal remedies. Mary was a battlefield nurse caring for the seriously wounded and dying soldiers on both sides of the conflict.

After the war, Mary returned to England in poor health and penniless. Her contribution to the soldiers would have gone unnoticed by the British people had it not been for a *London Times* correspondent named William Howard Russel. His story, describing her work on the battlefield, rescued her from bankruptcy.

Many scholars believe that Mary was not permitted to travel with Florence Nightingale to Crimea because of her age, race, and socioeconomic class. Mary, however, proved to be resourceful and did not accept "no" for an answer. She was confident in her skills and knew that she would be able to make a difference in the lives of the soldiers. She took every opportunity to learn. She valued the lessons her parents provided her, the stories the soldiers shared with her, and the experiences she had while running a boarding house.

In 1990, Mary was awarded with the Order of Merit by the Jamaican government, many years after her death. Mary Seacole's contributions were also recognized by the British people, and a memorial statue of her was placed on the grounds of Saint Thomas Hospital in London, opposite the Houses of Parliament.

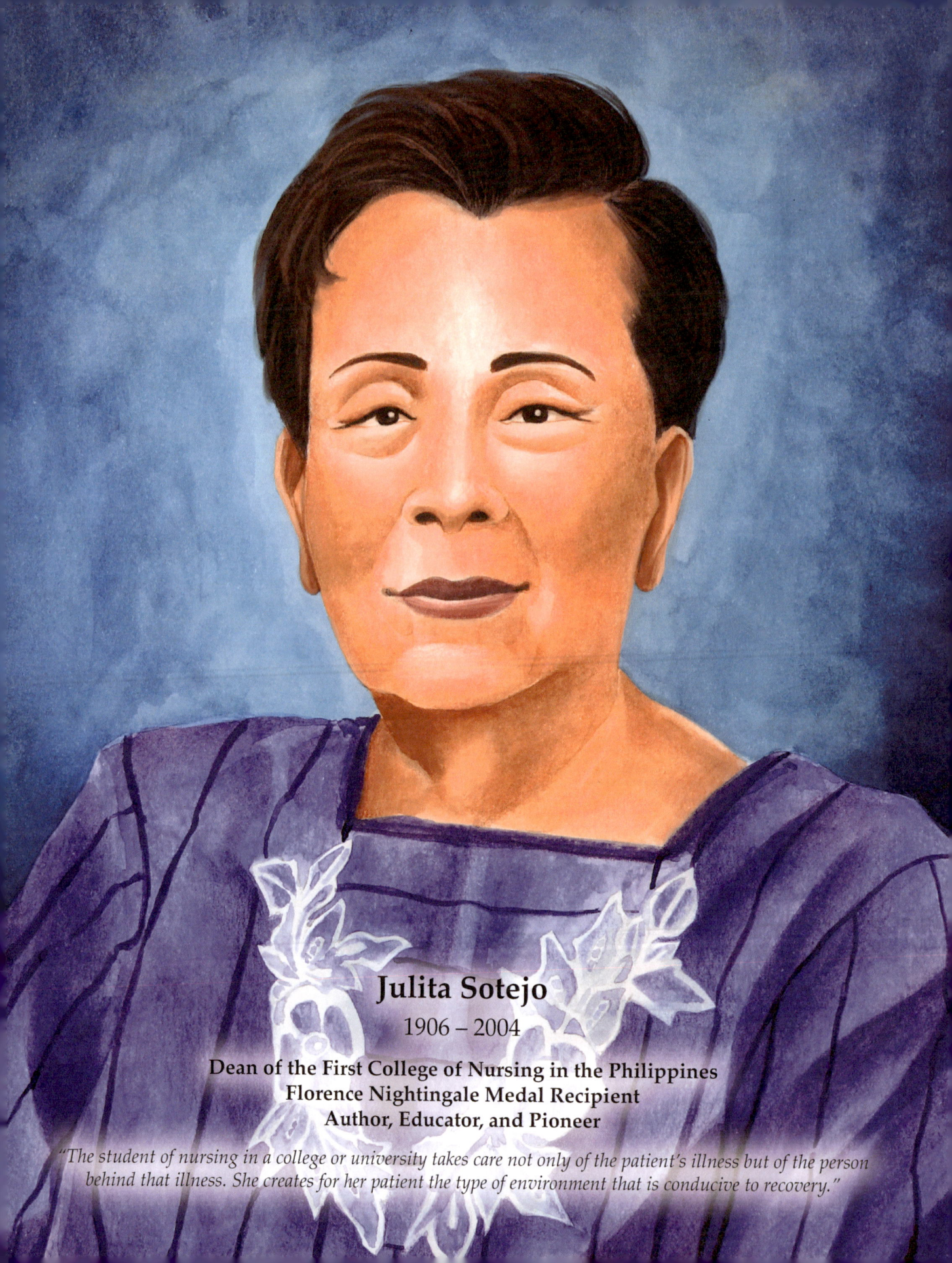

Julita Sotejo

1906 – 2004

Dean of the First College of Nursing in the Philippines
Florence Nightingale Medal Recipient
Author, Educator, and Pioneer

"The student of nursing in a college or university takes care not only of the patient's illness but of the person behind that illness. She creates for her patient the type of environment that is conducive to recovery."

Julita Villaruel Sotejo was born on June 16, 1906, in Gasan, Marinduque, when the Philippines was a United States colony. She was the eleventh child of Cenon and Margarita Sotejo. Julita was never able to know any of her older siblings. They all died before she was born due to childhood illnesses or epidemics that afflicted the island province. Julita attended high school in Boac, which was a distance from her home. Julita's father took her to Boac on Sunday afternoons in a horse-drawn carriage, called a calesa, and she stayed with family during the week. Cenon picked Julita up on Friday afternoons so they could be together as a family.

Julita hoped to become a lawyer but became a nurse so she could afford law school. She was admitted to the Philippine General Hospital School of Nursing in Manila. She was disappointed that as a new student, she and her classmates were assigned to care for patients in the wards before learning about their diseases in class. This did not prevent her from excelling, as she graduated as valedictorian in 1929. She was immediately recruited to teach at the school of nursing. Teaching by day, Julita attended law classes in the evenings. She achieved her goal by graduating as valedictorian from the Philippine Law School in 1936. She did not practice law, although she achieved the 6th highest score of all graduates on the Bar exam. She remained at the Philippine General Hospital School of Nursing as its principal.

Julita was a skilled leader, and she believed that to advance the profession of nursing in the Philippines, she needed additional education. The Rockefeller Foundation was interested in helping to improve the health conditions of people living in the Asia-Pacific, and it sponsored healthcare workers so they could study abroad. She was appointed Principal of the Philippine General Hospital School of Nursing in 1940 and was awarded a Rockefeller Foundation Fellowship. She studied in Toronto, Canada, and at the University of Chicago, earning a master's degree in nursing administration in 1943. Julita was unable to return home to the Philippines after graduation, as World War II was raging in the Pacific. She remained in Chicago, working as a clinical nurse at the Billings Hospital until June of 1945.

Julita returned to the Philippines to find her beloved Manila, the University of the Philippines, and the Philippines General Hospital in ruins. She resumed her role as principal at the school of nursing and joined her fellow nurses in anticipating a better life for their country. The Philippines were granted independence on July 4, 1946. Julita used the persuasion skills she learned in law school to implement the ideas from her master's thesis. After review and approval by the Philippine Nurses Association and the Board of Regents of the University of the Philippines, her goal of nurses being educated in a university had been achieved.

Nurse Sotejo became the first woman academic dean of the University of the Philippines. The 38 nursing students admitted in the first class studied both English and Spanish, world history, and social problems that affect health. One unique feature of the program was that the students chose their area of special study in their third year. Their education prepared them to be good leaders when they graduated.

Julita was the first President of the Philippine Nurses Association and founded the Academy of Nursing in the Philippines, the first research-oriented nursing association. In 1961, Nurse Julita Sotejo was awarded the highest international honor given to a nurse, the Florence Nightingale Medal, presented by the International Red Cross.

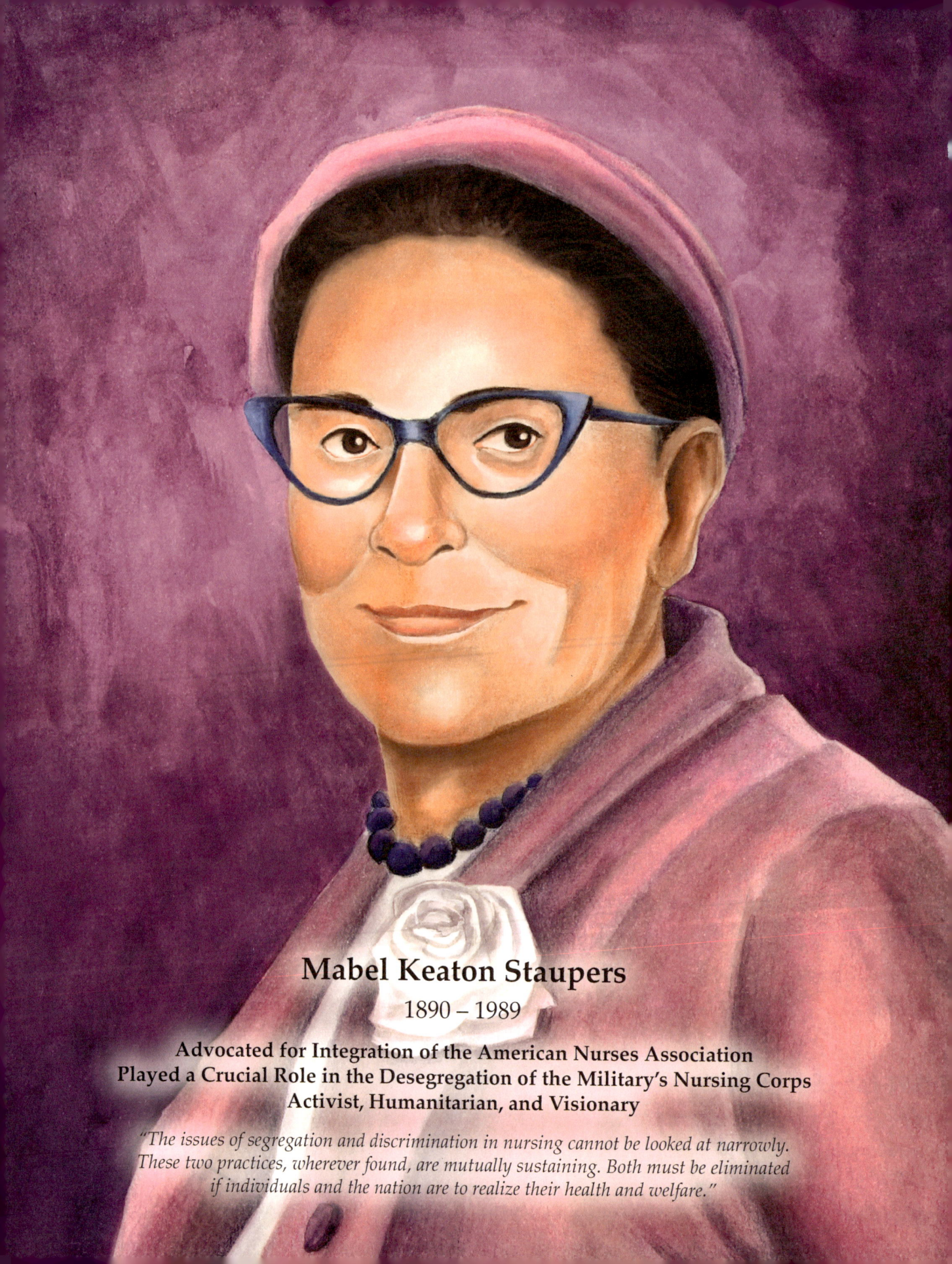

Mabel Keaton Staupers

1890 – 1989

**Advocated for Integration of the American Nurses Association
Played a Crucial Role in the Desegregation of the Military's Nursing Corps
Activist, Humanitarian, and Visionary**

*"The issues of segregation and discrimination in nursing cannot be looked at narrowly.
These two practices, wherever found, are mutually sustaining. Both must be eliminated
if individuals and the nation are to realize their health and welfare."*

Mabel Doyle was born on February 27, 1890, in Barbados, West Indies. She was born to Thomas and Pauline Doyle. Mable and her seamstress mother immigrated to New York City when she was 13 years old. Her father, who was a dentist, arrived in New York City a few years later. The year 1917 was an important one for Mabel, as she became a naturalized United States citizen and graduated with honors from the Freedom's Hospital School of Nursing in Washington, D.C. Shortly after graduation, Mabel married James Max Keaton. This marriage ended in divorce, but in 1931, she married Fritz C. Staupers, who supported her in her activism until his death in 1949.

Mabel worked as a private-duty nurse after graduation. She joined black doctors Louis T. Wright and James Wilson to create the Booker T. Washington Sanatorium. This was the first hospital in Harlem for black Americans; it was also the first hospital in New York that allowed black doctors to treat patients. Mabel was the director of nursing at this radical new hospital. She realized that in order to be influential in creating a better healthcare system for individuals in the black community, she would need to acquire additional education. Her next career move was to Philadelphia to pursue a working fellowship to study tuberculosis. Mabel returned to New York City in 1922, where she served as the executive secretary for the Harlem Tuberculosis Committee. Mabel was an extraordinary organizer known for her tireless energy, engaging sense of humor, and ability to bring different groups of people together.

Although Mabel experienced a great deal of professional success, she was deeply troubled by the racial discrimination she and members of the black community faced. Nursing schools were segregated, and the American Nurses Association (ANA) and the National League of Nursing Education, two of the most influential nursing organizations, did not accept black nurses living in 17 states, primarily those in the south.

Black Americans also had difficulty receiving medical care during this time. These injustices, which she witnessed daily, propelled Mabel to dedicate her life to improving the status of black nurses as well as promoting better healthcare for black Americans. In 1934, Mabel became the executive secretary of the National Association of Colored Graduate Nurses (NACGN), an organization founded by 52 nurses committed to promoting full integration of black female nurses into the nursing profession. (The term "colored "was used up until the 1970s to refer to black individuals. It is used here because that was the title of the organization at the time.)

Nurse Keaton Staupers was a woman who never let the word "no" get in the way of her achieving her mission. During World War II, she launched a campaign to encourage the integration of black nurses into the Armed Forces Nurse Corps. While black nurses were admitted, segregation remained. She was not discouraged. She met with First Lady Eleanor Roosevelt to decide the best course of action. Mabel led a nationwide letter-writing campaign and organized demonstrations of both black and white nurses to convince President Franklin D. Roosevelt to end segregation. On January 20, 1945, the War Department announced the end of racial quotas and discrimination. In 1948, the ANA announced full admission to black nurses, and the NACGN was disbanded.

Nurse Mabel Keaton Staupers was awarded the Spingarn Medal from the National Association for the Advancement of Colored People (NAACP) for her activism. Mabel captured her life's work in the autobiography *No Time for Prejudice: A Story of the Integration of Negroes in Nursing in the United States.*

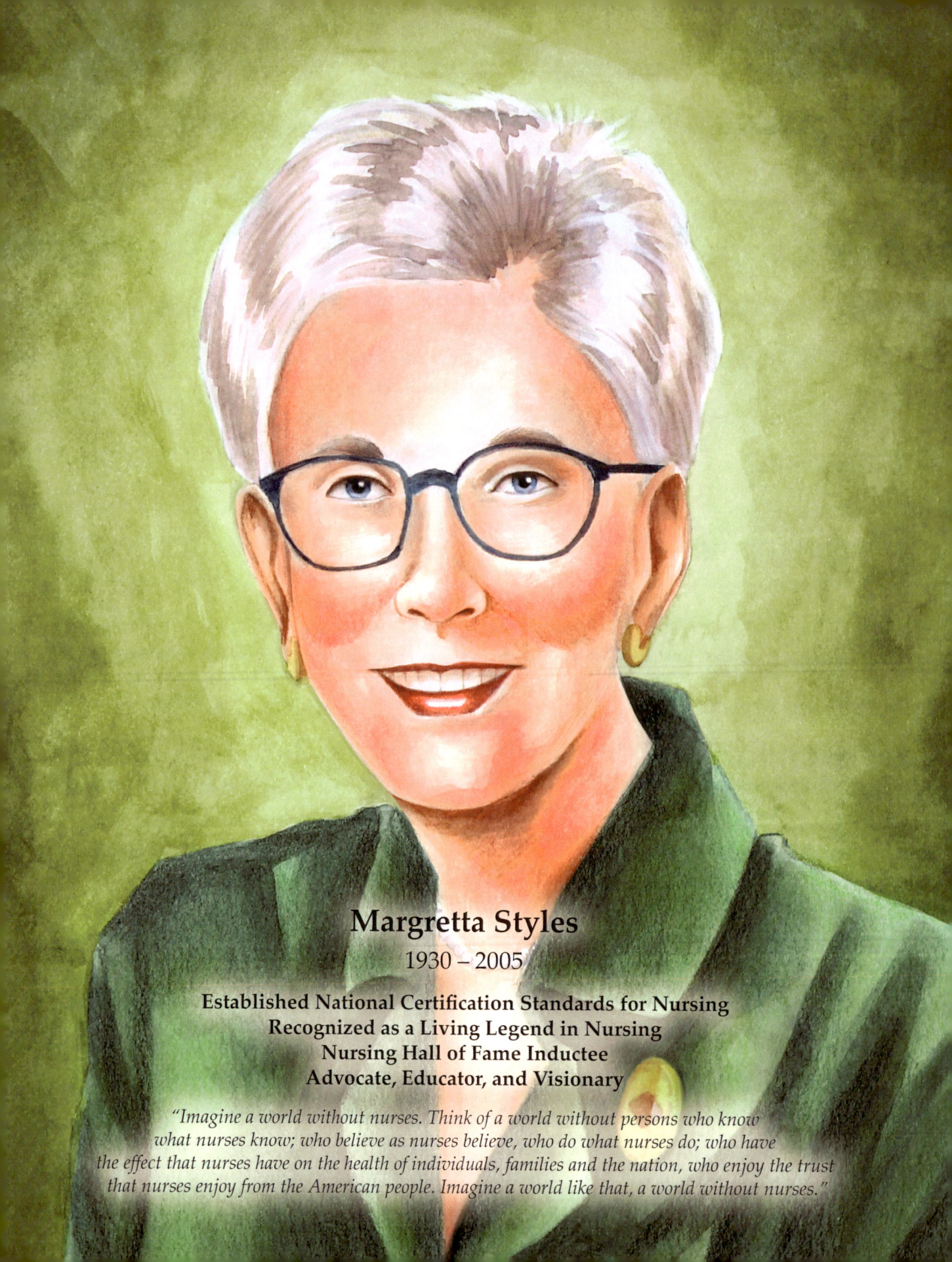

Margretta Styles

1930 – 2005

Established National Certification Standards for Nursing
Recognized as a Living Legend in Nursing
Nursing Hall of Fame Inductee
Advocate, Educator, and Visionary

"Imagine a world without nurses. Think of a world without persons who know what nurses know; who believe as nurses believe, who do what nurses do; who have the effect that nurses have on the health of individuals, families and the nation, who enjoy the trust that nurses enjoy from the American people. Imagine a world like that, a world without nurses."

Margretta Madden Styles, known as Gretta by all who knew and loved her, was a fascinating leader who advocated tirelessly for the profession of nursing. Gretta was born March 19, 1930, in Mount Union, Pennsylvania, the youngest of eight children. As a child, Gretta was curious and adventurous; she was flying a plane by herself over cornfields when she was just 16. Religion was very important to Gretta and her family. She considered entering the religious life and spent a year living in a convent in Puerto Rico after graduating from college. Since she held a bachelor's degrees in biology and chemistry, she was assigned to teach basic science classes in a school of nursing. She was an excellent teacher and found the sciences exciting and stimulating. Gretta decided to become a nurse and not to enter the convent.

Gretta earned a master's degree in nursing in 1954 from Yale as well as her doctorate in education from the University of Florida in 1968. While attending Yale, she met her husband, Doug, who was enrolled in the Episcopal Seminary. Doug supported her ambition during a time when most women were homemakers who dedicated themselves to parenting their children. She and Doug raised three children while she traveled the world, inspiring and teaching other nurse leaders.

Nurse Styles started her nursing career at the Veterans Administration Hospital in West Haven, Connecticut. Because of her intelligence, can-do attitude, and enthusiasm, new nurses sought her out. They knew Gretta had answers to their questions as well as the scientific reason for what they needed to do. Her dedication to nursing education led her to serve as dean at several nursing schools, including the University of Texas at San Antonio, Wayne State University, and University of California San Francisco.

Gretta always challenged herself to learn more, meet new people, and work with other professionals to advance nursing. One of her greatest dreams was to create a way for nurses to become credentialed. She wanted nurses to demonstrate their knowledge of a clinical specialty, just as doctors are required to do. She worked enthusiastically and tirelessly to create a testing system that showed the public and other professionals that nurses had specialized knowledge.

Nurse Styles was recognized as an expert, innovator, and leader and was elected to the National Academy of Medicine (NAM), an organization outside of the government that provides objective guidance on matters of medicine, technology, and health. One of Nurse Styles' greatest accomplishments was that she served as president of the American Nurses Association (ANA); the International Council of Nurses, representing nurses globally; and the American Nurses Credentialing Center (ANCC), which gives credentials to individual nurses in clinical specialties and gives credentials to hospitals that are known throughout the country for their excellence in patient care delivery.

Gretta was admired and respected because she was able to work with others to get things done. She inspired others to join her in moving her ideas forward. She was known to use the word "march" to let others know that she was moving forward with others by her side. In addition to her great leadership skills, Nurse Gretta Styles was also humble and expressed her gratitude to others often. Every year, the world's nurses celebrate "Certified Nurses Day" on March 19, the anniversary of her birth, to honor her and thank her for devoting her life to promoting the contributions of nurses everywhere.

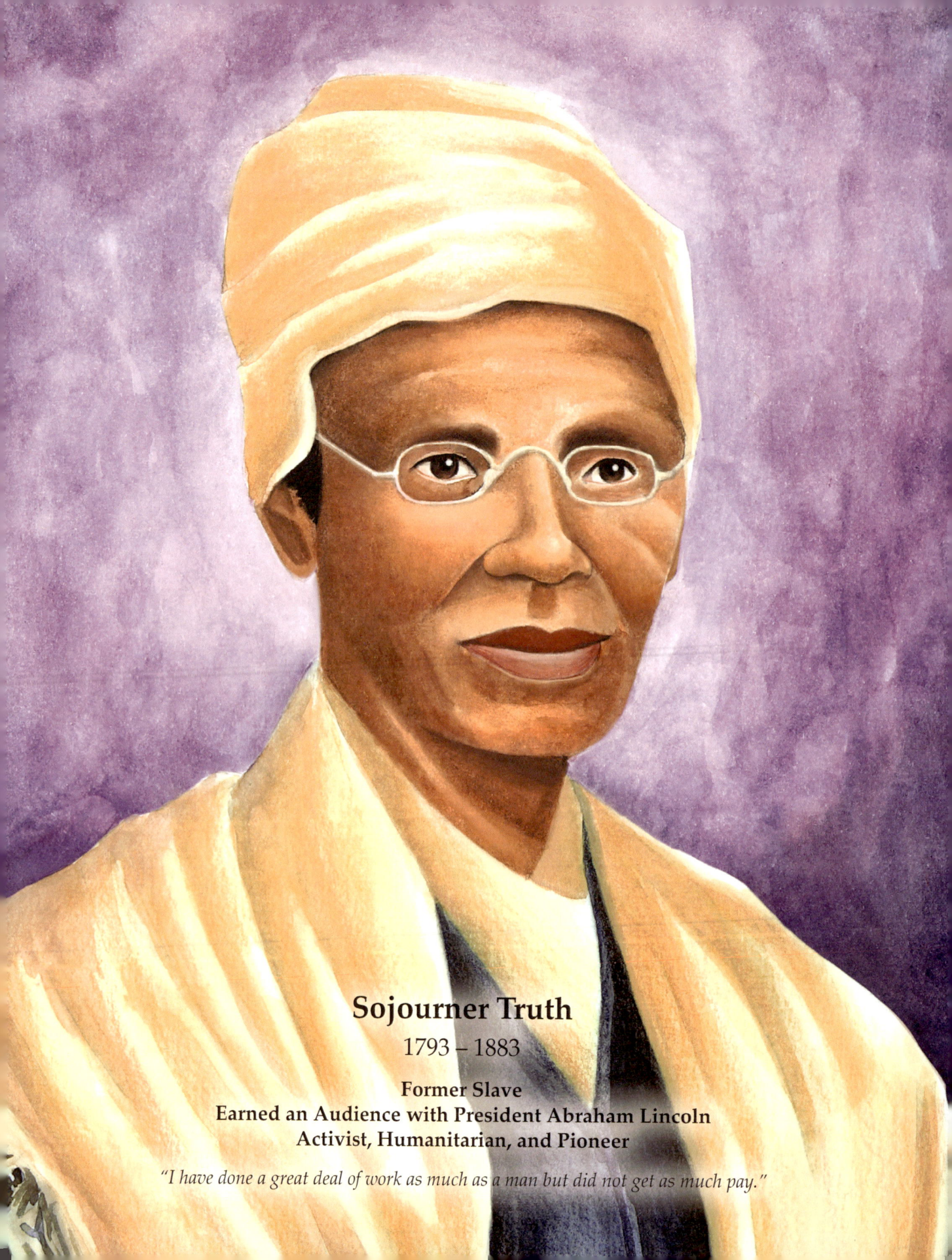

Sojourner Truth

1793 – 1883

Former Slave
Earned an Audience with President Abraham Lincoln
Activist, Humanitarian, and Pioneer

"I have done a great deal of work as much as a man but did not get as much pay."

Sojourner Truth's given name was Isabella Baumfree, and she was the youngest of twelve children born to Elizabeth and James Baumfree. Her parents were slaves on a plantation in northern New York. In the early 1800s, plantation owners bought and sold people to work on their farmlands. Isabella was born into slavery and was taken away from her family at the age of 9. She was sold for $100, along with a flock of sheep, to another family. At the age of 13, Isabella was sold to John Dumont and served as a nurse to his family. Isabella met Tom, another slave, and they had five children together, three daughters and two sons. James, the oldest child, died in infancy.

Tom and Isabella were promised freedom by Dumont, but he changed his mind when Isabella hurt her hand and could not work as hard. In 1826, Isabella escaped the plantation with her 5th child, Sophia. Tom chose not to leave and remained on the plantation with the other 4 children. A famous story written about Isabella's escape says that she walked away and did not run. She did not believe she had to run for her freedom; she simply decided to bravely walk away from a life that was not her own.

New York State passed the Anti-Slavery Law in 1827, one year after Isabella escaped the plantation. After slavery ended in New York, Dumont, her former slave owner, illegally sold her son Peter. Isabella sued the slave owner, and the United States Court ruled in Isabella's favor. Isabella was the first black woman to sue a white man and win. After becoming a free woman, Isabella moved to New York City and became a preacher, using her 6-feet tall frame and her powerful voice to teach, to encourage, and to inspire others. She renamed herself Sojourner Truth, a name that would match her personality at the pulpit.

Sojourner moved to Florence, Massachusetts, as the city became a northeastern center for the anti-slavery movement, also called abolitionism. Many former slaves bought homes in Florence and helped other slaves escape. This system of houses helping slaves escape was called the "Underground Railroad." Many abolitionists, like Frederick Douglass, traveled through Florence and advocated for Sojourner to speak at public forums, using her passion and energy to inspire others. Sojourner was able to support herself through her speaking engagements. She never learned to read or write, but she was able to dictate her autobiography, *The Narrative of Sojourner Truth*, to Olive Gilbert in 1850. In 1851, Sojourner made her most famous speech, *Ain't I a Woman*, at a Women's Rights Convention in Akron, Ohio. This speech argued that all women, no matter their race, should have rights equal to men.

The American Civil War began in 1861. Sojourner worked in Washington D.C. to recruit black soldiers and help organize relief programs to provide food, clothing, and supplies through the National Freedman's Relief Association. Sojourner advocated for nurse training programs. President Abraham Lincoln became aware of her work and invited her to the White House to meet with him. After the Civil War ended in 1865, Sojourner worked to find jobs for black soldiers and advocated for freed slaves to own land. She won another court case against a driver who physically tried to prevent her from riding a public streetcar because of the color of her skin.

Sojourner Truth eventually moved to Battle Creek, Michigan, and retired from public life with her daughters. For nearly thirty years, Sojourner was enslaved. She walked to freedom and dedicated her entire life to battling injustice.

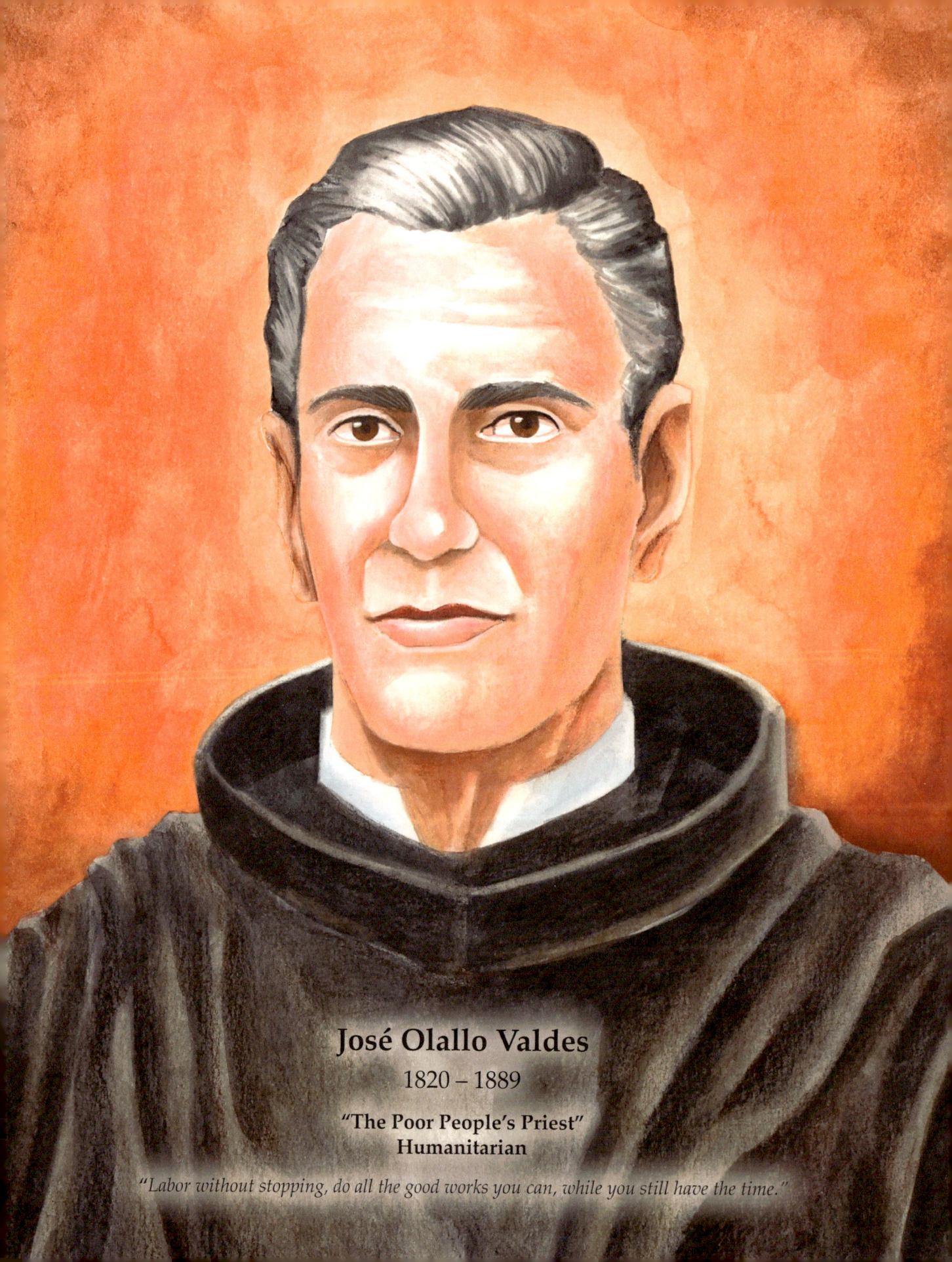

José Olallo Valdes

1820 – 1889

"The Poor People's Priest"
Humanitarian

"Labor without stopping, do all the good works you can, while you still have the time."

An unnamed baby boy was left at the Saint Joseph Orphanage in Havana, Cuba, with a note that said his date of birth was February 12, 1820. The caregivers in the orphanage named him José in honor of St. Joseph, Olallo in honor of the saint whose feast day he was born on, and Valdes in honor of the bishop of Havana. José lived and studied at a children's home and a charity house, and he received an excellent education, a luxury usually reserved for only the wealthy.

José was raised to be a thoughtful, kind, and responsible boy. At the age of 13, José entered the Hospitaller Order of St. John of God, the order of brothers who dedicated their lives to taking care of the sick and the poor. There were no nursing schools available when José entered religious life, so he learned how to be a nurse by watching the brothers care for the poor and enslaved. Two years later, José was transferred to the St. John of God Hospital in the city of Puerto Principe, now known as Camagüey, where he spent the rest of his life. He was known as Fray, or Friar Olallo. Fray Olallo cared for everyone who came to the hospital for help, including people with leprosy, cholera, and smallpox. It is said that in his 54 years of service to the sick, he only missed one night at the hospital.

During the Ten Years' War, also called the Great War, in which Cuba fought for its independence from Spain, José cared for soldiers from both sides of the conflict without judgement. The Spanish soldiers had taken control of the hospital, and José, without regard for his personal safety, defended the need for prisoners, orphans, elderly, and the war-wounded to be able to receive medical care. His act of courage gained him the respect of military authorities and prevented civil unrest that would have left many dead.

The Spanish army also prevented the Cuban people from practicing their religion. Most of the religious were evicted from Cuba, leaving Fray Olallo and another Brother in Camagüey. When that Brother died in 1876, José was left to care for the sick and carry on the mission of his order for 23 years all by himself.

Fray Olallo's compassion and kindness prompted the Archbishop of Santiago to encourage him to become a priest. Fray Olallo declined, as he was worried that he would have to stop caring for his beloved patients. He was given the nickname "Poor People's Priest" and was thereafter known as Father Olallo or Padre Olallo.

For 54 years, Padre Olallo lived and worked at St. John of God Hospital. He continued his nursing education by reading and teaching himself more advanced procedures. He even performed small surgeries. As money was scarce, he begged on the streets, using the donated funds for his patients. When the hospital could no longer afford a laundress, Padre Olallo washed his patients' clothes and bandages in the river.

On March 7, 1889, José died, and 2,000 of his countrymen attended his funeral. José Ollalo Valdes's reputation of holiness spread among the Cuban people, and many began to pray to him for help with their worries and suffering. José was beatified by Pope Benedict XVI, which is the first step in becoming a saint, after the recovery of a 3-year-old suffering from a rare cancer was deemed a miracle by the Roman Catholic Church. The family and friends of Daniela Cabera Ramos prayed to Padre Olalla for complete and instant healing, and their prayers were answered.

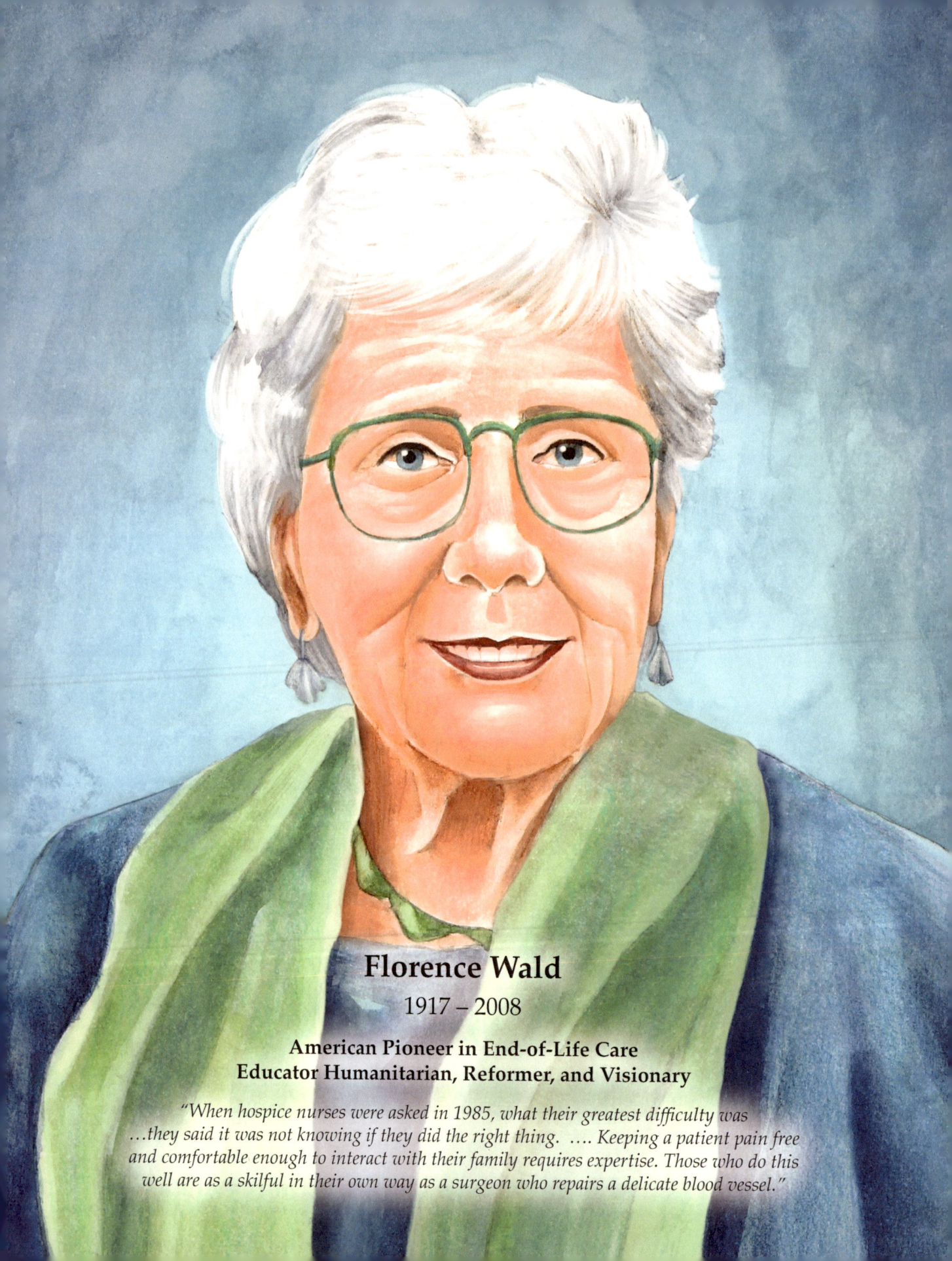

Florence Wald

1917 – 2008

**American Pioneer in End-of-Life Care
Educator Humanitarian, Reformer, and Visionary**

*"When hospice nurses were asked in 1985, what their greatest difficulty was
…they said it was not knowing if they did the right thing. …. Keeping a patient pain free
and comfortable enough to interact with their family requires expertise. Those who do this
well are as a skilful in their own way as a surgeon who repairs a delicate blood vessel."*

Florence Sophie Schorske Wald was born April 19, 1917, 13 days after the United States entered World War I. Florence's parents were immigrants from Germany who experienced a great deal of discrimination due to the U.S. and Germany being at war. Florence's parents did not have college degrees, but they were dedicated to reading and being well informed about world events. They passed this love of learning and curiosity on to their children. They spoke German in their home to encourage their children to be bilingual; however, Florence and her brother feared being rejected by other children, so they chose to speak English instead.

Florence was often sick as a child and was hospitalized on several occasions. During one hospital stay, Florence was put in quarantine. She had to be in a room by herself, and her family could not visit her because she had scarlet fever, a contagious disease. Florence was frightened and felt alone. It was her private-duty nurse who cared for her, made her feel safe, and offered comfort. It was during her time in the hospital that Florence learned about the skill and compassion that nurses provide, and she decided to become a nurse. Although her parents valued education, Florence's father did not believe women needed to attend college. Her mother and brother were able to change his mind. Florence graduated from Mount Holyoke College and then received a master's degree in nursing from Yale.

She began her career at Children's Hospital in Boston, then moved to New York to work at the Henry Street Settlement, which provided nursing care to the poor. Florence believed passionately that nurses should be dedicated to treating the "whole person" from birth to death.

In 1944, Florence shocked her family and joined the United States Army Signal Corps. When World War II ended, Florence left the military and returned to nursing. She earned a master's degree in psychiatric nursing from Yale and eventually became Dean of the School of Nursing at Yale. Nurse Wald encouraged nurses to be curious and conduct research. She also renewed her friendship with a man who had proposed to her years earlier. His name was Henry Wald, and he was a widower with two small children. He read about Florence's appointment in the newspaper and contacted her; they were married a year later.

Inspired by the work of Dame Cicely Saunders, from the United Kingdom who was planning the world's first hospice, Florence went to London to work at St. Christopher's Hospice. Florence learned as much as she could to prepare for opening the first Hospice in the U.S., and she educated nurses and doctors about caring for the dying. Hospice care was not practiced in the United States. Often, death was viewed as a failure. Doctors did not want to take hope away from their patients, so they did not always tell patients that there was no other treatment that would keep them alive.

Nurse Wald led the movement to improve care of the dying. In 1974, she opened the first in-home Hospice in Connecticut. Six years later, she founded a Hospice where the dying could be cared for by their loved ones and receive assistance from the staff skilled in care of the dying. Today, there are over 5,500 Hospices in the U.S.

Nurse Florence Wald held on to her beliefs of social justice, compassion, and dignity, and she changed the way the terminally ill are cared for in this country. She led by example, and at the age 91, she died peacefully at home, surrounded by her family.

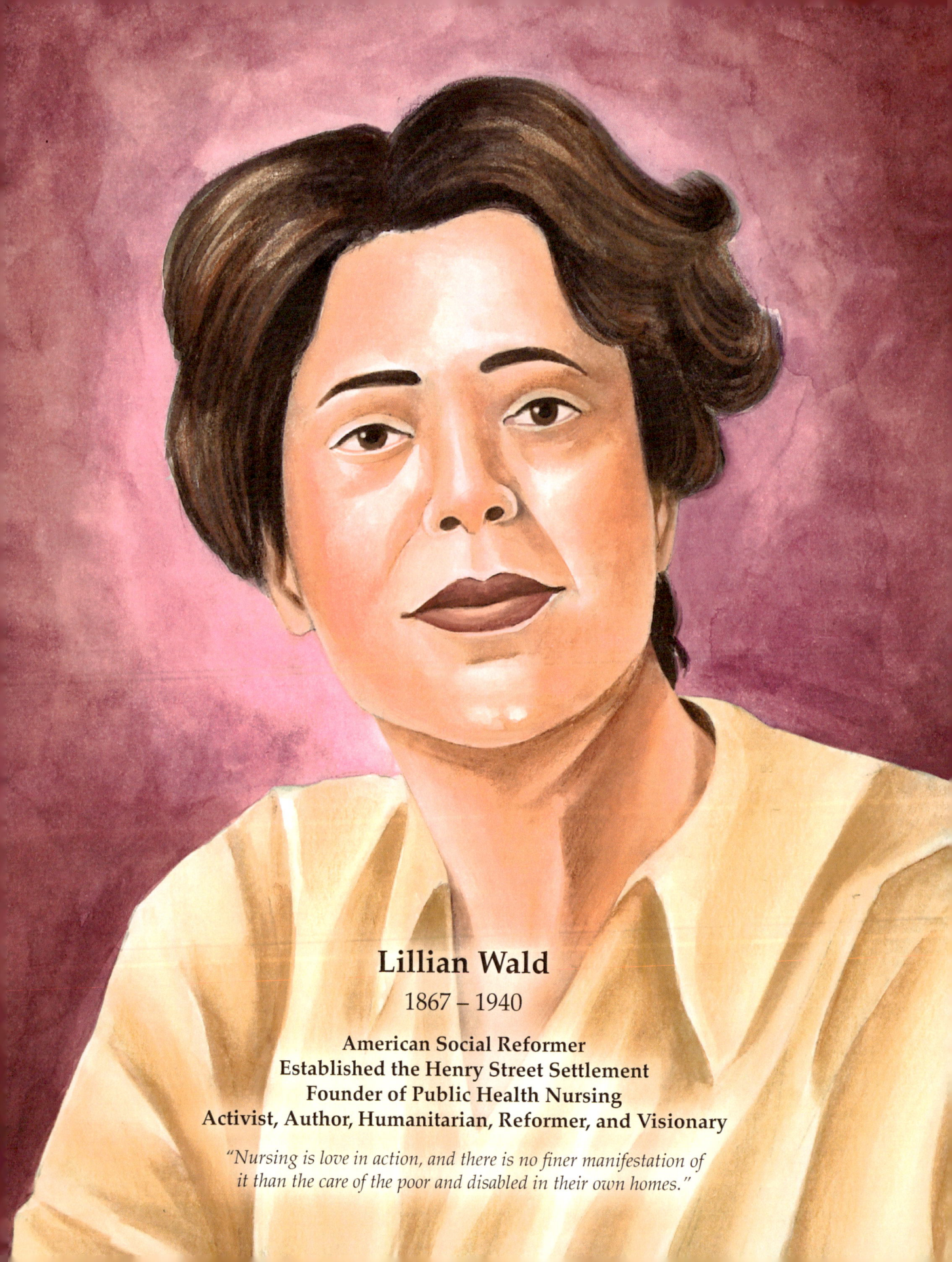

Lillian Wald

1867 – 1940

American Social Reformer
Established the Henry Street Settlement
Founder of Public Health Nursing
Activist, Author, Humanitarian, Reformer, and Visionary

"Nursing is love in action, and there is no finer manifestation of it than the care of the poor and disabled in their own homes."

Lillian D. Wald was born in Cincinnati, Ohio, on March 10, 1867. She was the third of four children born to Max and Minnie Schwarz Wald, who immigrated from Germany. Lillian's father was a successful businessman who sold eyeglass goods. He moved the family to Rochester when Lillian was 11 years old. Lillian and her siblings were lucky to grow up in a loving and happy family, and they had everything they needed or wanted. Lillian was an outstanding student and excelled in the arts, math, and science. She also had a natural ability for foreign languages. At the age of 16, Lillian applied to Vassar College but was rejected because they considered her too young. Lillian was restless and felt restricted by the limited options for women; she was seeking a purpose for her life. Then she met a nurse, and her future seemed clear.

Julia, Lillian's older sister, was pregnant and became ill while Lillian was visiting her. A trained nurse from Bellevue Hospital was sent to care for Julia. Lillian, never having encountered a nurse before, was impressed with the excellent care she provided. She decided at that moment that nursing would provide her with the purpose in life she was seeking. In 1889, Lillian applied to the New York Hospital's School of Nursing and entered her older sister's birthdate on the application to make sure she would not be rejected again because of her age.

At the time that Lillian chose to enter nursing school, nursing was considered "women's work" and had low status as an occupation. Nursing care, before the Crimean and Civil Wars, was carried out by women in religious orders or those from lower-class homes who received no more than 35 cents a day. However, the world was changing, as women were demanding it. After graduation in 1891, Lillian began working in an institution that provided care to children with mental illnesses. She left after a year, frustrated by her inability to make a difference. She enrolled in the Women's Medical College of the New York Infirmary, thinking that becoming a doctor would give her more authority to improve the care of children and the poor. While she found the classes interesting, she decided a career in medicine was not for her.

Lillian began teaching immigrants at the Jewish Sabbath School on Henry Street. One day, a young girl ran into Lillian's class, pleading for help for her sick mother. Lillian accompanied the girl back to her home and encountered the gravely ill mother, who was lying in blood-soaked sheets after having given birth two days earlier. Lillian cared for the mother and was overcome by the family's poor living conditions. She now realized her purpose. She would bring nurses into the homes of the poor so the nurses could see firsthand what each person needed. This was the beginning of the "public health nurse."

Nurse Wald began her crusade for the poor by using her talents to get funding to create the Henry Street Settlement, a place which offered social services, opportunities for the arts, health and nutrition classes, and a playground for children. By 1913, the Settlement had expanded to seven buildings on Henry Street and two other locations in the city, offering its services to thousands needing help. Lillian was an activist and a peacemaker who led reforms for social justice, public health, child labor laws, safe housing, and decent living wages. She helped create the Federal Children's Bureau in 1912.

Nurse Lillian Wald understood the social causes of poverty and dedicated her life to eliminating them. She made the world better.

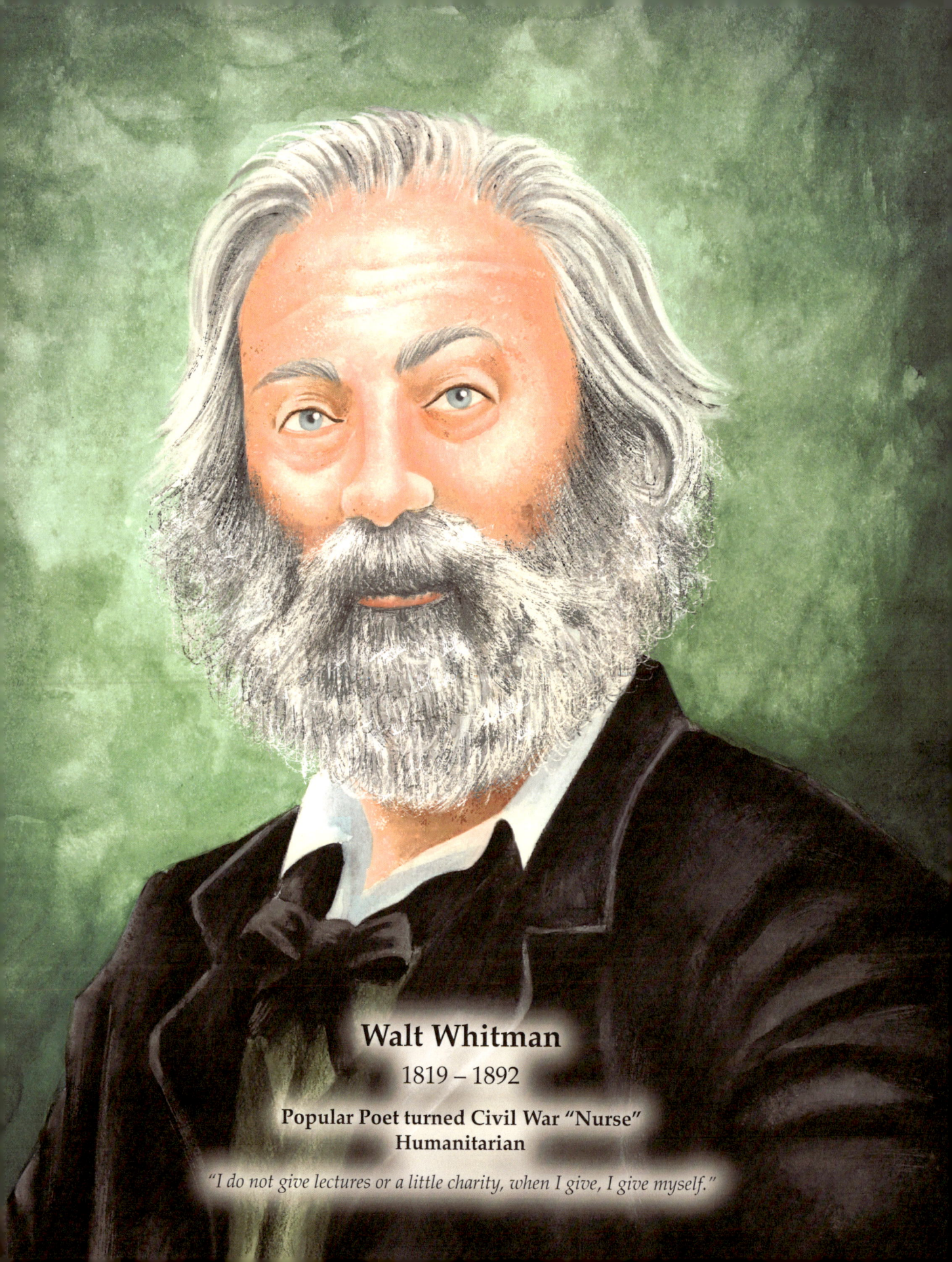

Walt Whitman

1819 – 1892

Popular Poet turned Civil War "Nurse"
Humanitarian

"I do not give lectures or a little charity, when I give, I give myself."

Walt Whitman, one of America's greatest poets, was born on May 31, 1819, in West Hills, New York, the second of nine children. His father was a house builder, and his mother was a homemaker. He grew up poor and left school at 11 to help support his family. He loved to read and began to write poetry as a young boy. When he was 12, he started working at a printing press, and throughout his younger years, he worked at various newspapers in New York City as a printer, editor, and writer. At 17, he became a teacher in a one-room schoolhouse after a devastating fire destroyed the publishing building.

Throughout his young life, he met political greats such as Martin Van Buren, the 8th United States President, along with famous poets, the most notable being Ralph Waldo Emerson, who became an admirer of Whitman's work. *Leaves of Grass*, one of Whitman's most famous works, was published before he began his work as a volunteer nurse in the Civil War.

In April of 1861, the American Civil War began, and Walt's younger brother enlisted in the Union Army. While his brother was fighting, Whitman visited injured soldiers in many New York City war hospitals. When Walt saw the name of his brother among the injured in the war in the newspaper, he traveled to find his brother in Virginia. Fortunately, his brother was not seriously wounded, but Whitman was shocked by what he saw on the battlefield. He moved to Washington D.C., took a low-paying job in the Army Paymaster's Office as a clerk, and began volunteering to care for the soldiers.

There was no formal training for nurses during the Civil War. Walt learned to nurse by watching others care for injured soldiers. He spent his free time in the hospitals, tending to the needs of the wounded and dying, and spent his own money so he could bring food, candy, writing paper, and pencils to the soldiers. He sat with the fatally wounded during their final hours of life. By listening to their stories, acknowledging their anxieties, and offering his presence, Walt helped reduce the soldiers' fear and suffering. Whitman estimated that he took care of 80,000 soldiers during the 3 years he volunteered at the hospitals.

He was so inspired, so he continued to write his poetry to reflect the war times. *Drum-Taps,* the poetry collection he wrote during this time, is considered a masterpiece, capturing the intensity and array of emotions Walt experienced from the beginning of the Civil War to its end. His words convey empathy and compassion, fear and terror, and kindness and humanity masterfully. The experiences he describes create a picture so real and vivid that the reader of his words is on the Virginia battlefields, seeing what he saw, hearing what he heard, and feeling what he felt.

After the Civil War, Whitman accepted another government position. He had gained popularity as a poet and was getting ready to publish his famed *Drum-Taps*. He postponed the release of this poetry collection when he learned of President Lincoln's assassination. Walt was heartbroken by Lincoln's death and wrote poems that showed his admiration for the slain president. *"When Lilacs Last in the Dooryard Bloom'd"* and *"O Captain! My Captain!"* were the two poems added to his wartime tribute.

During his lifetime, Walt held many different jobs, traveled the country, and met many people. His many literary works reflect his complicated life. While he never formally trained as a nurse, Walt Whitman tended to the wounded, collecting their stories and healing their bodies.

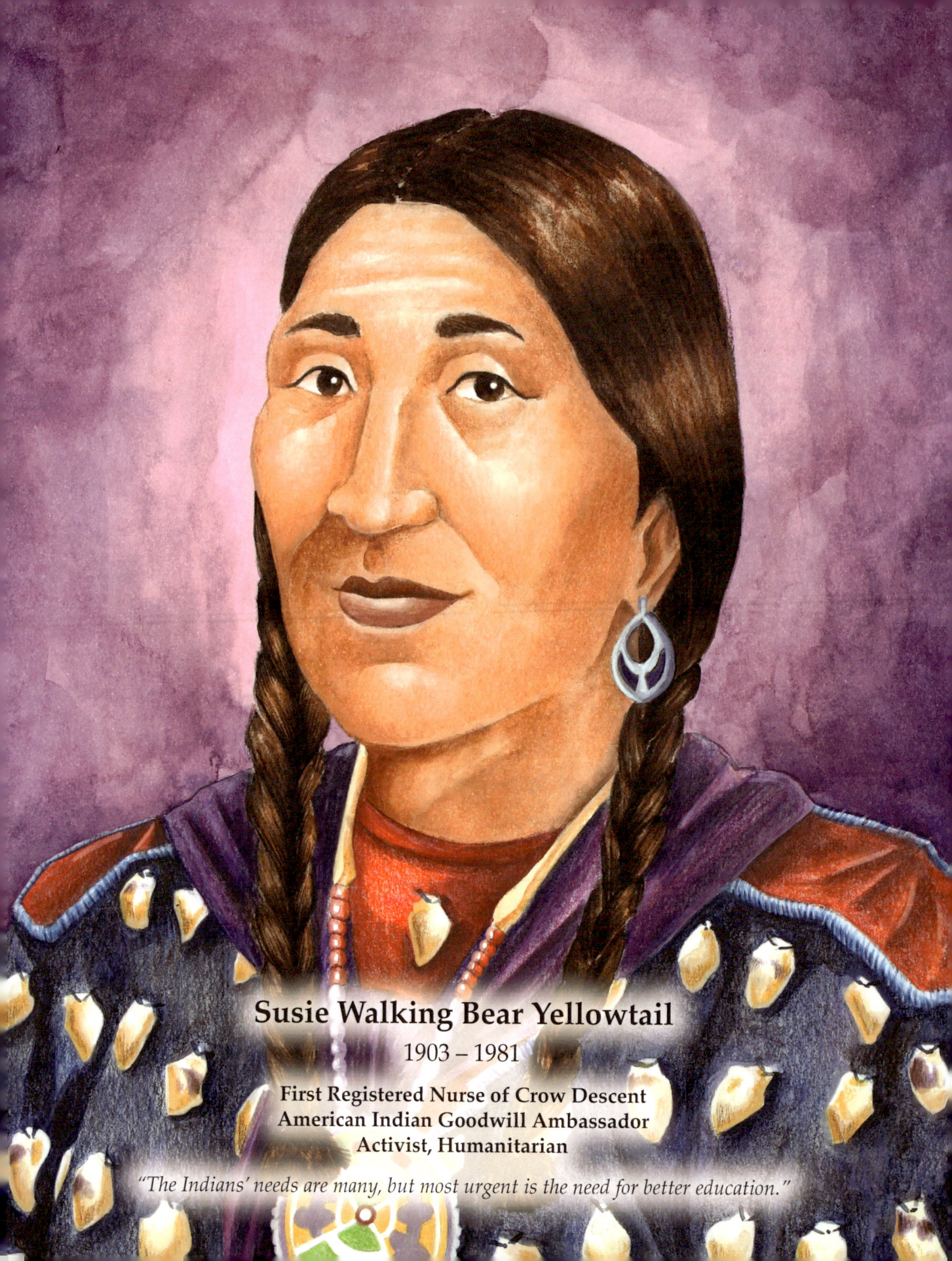

Susie Walking Bear Yellowtail

1903 – 1981

First Registered Nurse of Crow Descent
American Indian Goodwill Ambassador
Activist, Humanitarian

"The Indians' needs are many, but most urgent is the need for better education."

Susie Walking Bear was an American Indian born to the Apsáalooke (Crow) tribe in Montana in 1903. She was orphaned at the age of 12 and was sent to a boarding school on the reservation. She learned the traditional American Indian way of life, including the Apsáalooke language, values, and culture, while beginning to learn English at the boarding school. The blending of the two cultures remained with her as she attended schools in Oklahoma and Massachusetts. Susie graduated with honors from the Boston City Hospital's School of Nursing in 1923 and became the first United States registered nurse of Apsáalooke heritage.

Susie dedicated her nursing career to her American Indian people. She worked as a private-duty and homecare nurse on various reservations in Oklahoma and Minnesota. In 1929, Walking Bear returned to the Apsáalooke reservation in Montana and married Tom Yellowtail, a tribal and spiritual leader. She and Tom raised three children and took in many other children from the reservation who were in need.

Susie Walking Bear Yellowtail used her knowledge of Indian culture and her nursing knowledge to improve the health of American Indians. For centuries, American Indians have been granted fewer privileges than other citizens. During the last 300 years, land rights were taken away from American Indians, forcing them to live on reservations with very few resources available. Opportunities for education and quality healthcare remain limited. Living on American Indian reservations could mean that hospitals were thousands of miles away, living conditions were poor, and the opportunities for regular doctor and nurse visits were not available. Susie worked for the Bureau of Indian Affairs on the reservation and saw firsthand the healthcare injustices the American Indian people suffered. Susie realized that she would have to advocate for healthcare justice for American Indians for the rest of her life.

Walking Bear Yellowtail traveled to reservations all over the country to learn about the healthcare needs of her people and correct the injustices they faced. Susie took notes and kept records of how American Indian children were dying as their mothers carried them on their backs, walking twenty miles to get medical attention. She spoke about the differences in cultures that prevented doctors and nurses from understanding their tribal healing practices. She alerted legislators about unethical procedures that were being performed on women in her community. Susie advocated for healthcare reform and worked tirelessly to improve the living conditions on the reservations. She worked in the U.S. Public Health Service and on the Montana Advisory Committee. She acted as a Goodwill Ambassador to foreign countries and was appointed to the Public Health, Education, and Welfare Board.

Susie was respected by world leaders for her passion, determination, and devotion to her people. She was awarded the U.S. President's Award for Outstanding Nursing Care in 1962. She continued her advocacy for improved education, safety, and healthcare for American Indians through various boards, committees, and councils. Susie worked with many United States presidents to promote the health of the American Indian people.

Susie was proud of her heritage and never missed an opportunity to teach others about her tribe's history, culture, and contributions. Susie formed the American Indian Nurses Association; in 1978, she was named "Grandmother of American Indian Nurses." She is also called "Bright Morning Star" by members of the Crow tribe. Nurse Susie Walking Bear Yellowtail dedicated her life to reducing the suffering of her people, and she encouraged others in her community to become nurses and continue the work she started. There remains much work to be done!

SOURCE NOTES

Nightingale, Florence

p. 14 *"When I am…work of my life."* The Public Domain Review. The Voice of Florence Nightingale. 2009. https://www.publicdomainreview.org/collections/the voice-of-florence-nightingale.

Abdellah, Faye

p. 18 *"We cannot wait…has been completed."* https://www.newswise.com/articles/dr-faye-g-abdellah-founding-dean-of-daniel-k-inouye-graduate-school-of-nursing-dies-at-97.

Al-Aslamia, Rufaida

p. 20 *"We want to…as we can."* Kolleen Miller-Rosser, Ysanne Chapman, Karen Francis. Historical, cultural, and contemporary influences on the status of women in nursing in Saudi Arabia (July 19, 2006), *The Online Journal of Issues in Nursing (OJIN) 11(3).*

Barton, Clara

p. 22 *"I may be…and nurse them."* Elizabeth Brown Pryor. *Clara Barton: Professional Angel* (Philadelphia: University of Pennsylvania Press, 1987). p. 80.

Blake, Florence Guiness

p. 24 *"The nurse needs…cope with stress."* http://videos.med.wisc.edu/videos/2896.

Bradley, Ruby

p. 26 *"The question is…in life again."* https://www.appalachianhistory.net/2018/11/hometown-wisdom-in-time-of-war.html.

p. 26 *"It was all…a day's work."* https://www.identifymedals.com/article/why-colonel-ruby-bradley-was-known-as-the-angel-in-fatigues/.

Breckinridge, Mary

p. 28 "Work for children…their loving hearts." https://www.proedcenter.com/working-with-children-before-born/.

Callen, Maude

p. 30 *"I've seen people…a better life."* https://twoleavessametree.blogspot.com/2013/08/midwife-monday-maude-callen.html.

Carnegie, Mary Elizabeth

p. 32 *"The story of…of human beings."* Van Betten, and Melisa Moriarty. *Nursing Illuminations: A Book of Days.* (St. Louis: Mosby, 2004) p. 231.

Cavell, Edith

p. 34 *"Patriotism is not…bitterness towards anyone."* Van Betten, and Melisa Moriarty. *Nursing Illuminations: A Book of Days.* (St. Louis: Mosby, 2004) p. 709.

Christman, Luther

p. 36 *"Many of the…education among nurses."* Beth P. Houser and Kathy N. Houser. *Pivotal Moments in Nursing Moments. Volume 1.* (Indianapolis: Sigma Theta Tau, 2004). p. 78.

Clifford, Joyce

p. 38 *"I believe strongly…improve patient care."* https://www.mghpcs.org/caring/Assets/documents/issues/2006/May_25_2006%20Nurse%20Week.pdf.

Cooper, Signe

p. 40 *"Each person has…the next generation."* https://news.wisc.edu/nursing-pioneer-signe-skott-cooper-from-the-farm-to-the-battlefield/.

DeLellis, Saint Camillus

p. 42 *"More love in those hands brother."* http://www.orderofstcamillus.ie/st-camillus.

Diers, Donna

p. 44 *"Nurse is not…most fascinated companion."* Donna Diers. *Speaking of Nursing.* (Sudbury: Jones Bartlett, 2004). p. 178.

p. 44 *"Nurses deal with…without even asking."* Donna Diers and David Evans. Excellence in Nursing. *Journal of Nursing Scholarship.* 1980, 12(2). p. 27.

Dix, Dorothea

p. 46 *"I appear as…oppressed and desolate."* David Forrester (Ed.) *Nursing's Greatest Leaders: A History of Activism.* (New York: Springer, 2016). p. 176.

Dorr, Anita

p. 48 *"We felt that…to help ourselves."* Kendra Mims. First foot forward. ENA Connection. 2015, 39(4) p. 10.

Dumas, Rhetaugh

p. 50 *"From infancy I…welfare of others."* https://www.chicagotribune.com/news/ct-xpm-2007-07-28-0707270827-story.html.

p. 50 *"I accepted President…to be here."* As quoted by Joyce J. Fitzpatrick, remark made at conference by R. Dumas.

Ferguson, Vernice

p. 52 *"What is good…for the girls."* Beth P. Houser and Kathy N. Houser. *Pivotal Moments in Nursing Moments. Volume 1.* (Indianapolis: Sigma Theta Tau, 2004). p. 97.

Goodrich, Annie

p. 54 *"Knowledge is more… it is responsibility."* Van Betten, and Melisa Moriarty. *Nursing Illuminations: A Book of Days.* (St. Louis: Mosby, 2004). p. 155.

Henderson, Virginia

p. 56 *"The unique function…rapidly as possible."* https://www.currentnursing.com/nursing_theory/Henderson.html.

Ibuka, Yae

p. 58 *"Father it is…and work here."* Quoted and translated by Ikuno Yamaguchi, President of Japan Catholic Nurses Association, personal correspondence Joselyn Modic Banda.

p. 58 *"Exceptional courage and…or nursing education."* https://www.identifymedals.com/article/florence-nightingale-the-life-and-medals-of-the-lady-with-the-lamp/.

Johnson-Brown, Hazel

p. 60 *"Positive progress towards…you will have."* https://www.encyclopedia.com/education/news-wires-white-papers-and-books/johnson-hazel-1927.

p. 60 *"Never have and never will."* http://www.chestercohistorical.org/historys-people-hazel-johnson-brown-first-female-black-general.

Kelly, Kious

p. 62 *"Unfortunately, in many…alter the experience."* https://health.mountsinai.org/blog/helping-a-family-through-a-difficult-journey/.

Kenny, Sister Elizabeth

p. 64 *"Panic plays no…of a nurse."* Martha Ostens. *And They Shall Walk: The Story of Sister Elizabeth Kenny.* (New York: Dodd Mead, 1943). p. 23.

King, Susie Taylor

p. 66 *"It seems strange…sympathy and pity."* Van Betten, and Melisa Moriarty. *Nursing Illuminations: A Book of Days.* (St. Louis: Mosby, 2004). p. 459.

Lane, Sharon

p. 68 *"Finally got my…can go sooner."* Phillip Bigler. *Hostile Fire: The Life and Death of First Lieutenant Sharon Lane.* (Arlington: Vandamere Press, 1996). p. 72.

Leininger, Madeline

p. 70 **"Why in the world…to their culture?"** https://www.youtube.com/watch?v=a4GTo_uthZQ.

p. 70 *"Well that is…you to discover."* Madeline Leninger. *Culture Care Diversity and Universality.* (Burlington: Jones and Bartlett, 2001). p. 21.

Mahoney, Mary Eliza

p. 72 *"Work more and…the previous year."* https://www.govtrack.us/congress/bills/109/hconres386/text/e.

Maxwell, Anna

p. 74 *"The pioneers of…instructed nurses."* Van Betten, and Melisa Moriarty. *Nursing Illuminations: A Book of Days.* (St. Louis: Mosby, 2004). p. 155.

Mayer, Schwester Selma

p. 76 *"Because I lost…profession of nursing."* https://www.ifcj.org/news/fellowship-blog/nurse-selma-2/.

Moreno, Jennifer

p. 78 *"Be strong when…you are victorious."* https://www.facebook.com/MadiganHealth/videos/2135523143368274/.

Mother Teresa

p. 80 *"The biggest disease…deserted by everybody."* Elizabeth Knowles (Ed). As quoted in *The Oxford Dictionary of Quotations.* (Oxford: Oxford Press: 2014). p. 768.

p. 80 *"To serve the…shunned by everyone."* https://mtctampa.org/mother-teresa-of-calcutta/.

p. 80 *"I have lived…of an angel."* https://m.rediff.com/news/mother/teresa.htm.

Nutting, Adelaide

p. 82 *"We need to…only working power."* Van Betten, and Melisa Moriarty. *Nursing Illuminations: A Book of Days.* (St. Louis: Mosby, 2004). p. 645.

Peplau, Hildegard

p. 84 *"Nurses are available…the health services."* Hildegard Peplau. *Interpersonal Relations in Nursing.* (New York: Putnam, 1952). p. 16.

Reinmann, Christiane

p. 86 *"When I decided…not a lady."* https://www.workingnurse.com/articles/Christiane-Reimann-and-the-International-Council-of-Nurses.

Robb, Isabel Hampton

p. 88 *"Nurses are trusted…other human beings."* https://magazine.nursing.jhu.edu/2010/11/more-than-stethoscopes-and-blood-pressure-cuffs/.

Rogers, Lina

p. 90 *"A sensible school…of a community."* https://www.workingnurse.com/articles/lina-rogers-the-first-school-nurse.

Rogers, Martha

p. 92 *"Nursing's story is…into human service."* Van Betten, and Melisa Moriarty. *Nursing Illuminations: A Book of Days.* (St. Louis: Mosby, 2004). p. 277.

Saunders, Dame Cicely

p. 94 *"You matter because…until you die."* https://hospice-vic.org/hospice/honoring-the-legacy-of-cecily-saunders-founder-of-modern-hospice/.

p. 94 *"As the body…spirit becomes stronger."* https://metro.co.uk/2018/06/22/meet-dame-cicely-saunders-humanitarian-transformed-end-life-care-hospice-7650960/#:~:text=Her%20thinking%20was%20that%20'as,the%20end%20of%20your%20life.

p. 94 *"You matter because…of your life."* https://www.stchristophers.org.uk/home-2-2/about/.

Seacole, Mary

p. 96 *"I trust that…her illustrious dead."* https://blogs.canterbury.ac.uk/library/wonderful-adventures-of-mary-seacole/.

Sotejo, Julita

p. 98 *"The student of nursing…conducive to recovery."* Quoted and reported by Luz Tungpalan, former Dean School of Nursing, University of Philipines, personal correspondence Mary Beth Modic.

Staupers, Mabel Keaton

p. 100 *"The issues of…health and welfare."* Van Betten, and Melisa Moriarty. *Nursing Illuminations: A Book of Days.* (St. Louis: Mosby, 2004). p. 121.

Styles, Margretta

p. 102 *"Imagine a world…world without nurses."* https://grettafoundation.org/who-we-are/our-mission-history/.

Truth, Sojourner

p. 104 *"I have done…as much pay."* https://spartacus-educational.com/USAStruth.htm.

Valdes, Jose Ollalo

p. 106 *"Labor without stopping…have the time."* https://todayscatholic.org/wp-content/uploads/pdf-archives/2008/45Dec%2C7%2C2008.pdf.

Wald, Florence

p. 108 *"When hospice nurses…delicate blood vessel."* Van Betten, and Melisa Moriarty. *Nursing Illuminations: A Book of Days.* (St. Louis: Mosby, 2004). p. 229.

Wald, Lillian

p. 110 *"Nursing is love…their own homes."* https://www.nahc.org/wp-content/uploads/2017/10/Remembering-Lillian-Wald.pdf.

Whitman, Walt

p. 112 *"I do not…I give myself."* Van Betten, and Melisa Moriarty. *Nursing Illuminations: A Book of Days.* (St. Louis: Mosby, 2004). p. 312.

Yellowtail, Susie Walking Bear

p. 114 *"The Indians' needs…for better education."* https://mhs.mt.gov/Portals/11/education/Montanans/yellowtail2.pdf.

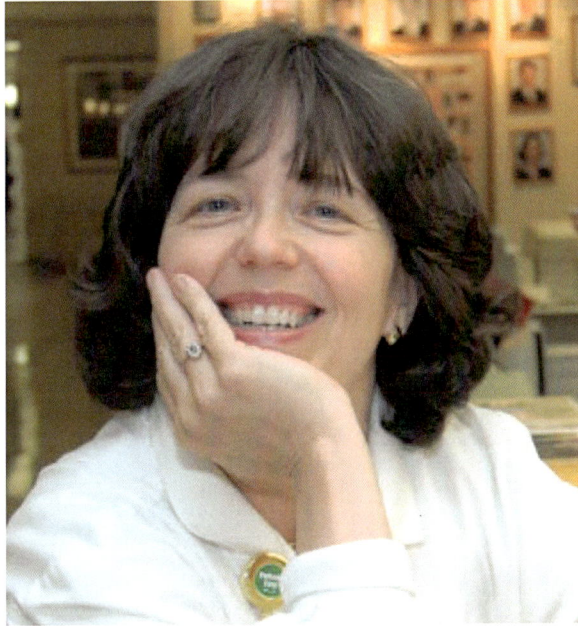

Mary Beth Modic, DNP, APRN-CNS, CDCES, FAAN is a Clinical Nurse Specialist and Certified Diabetes Care and Education Specialist. She loves being a nurse and teaching people with diabetes how to take the best care of themselves so they can remain healthy. She, along with Dr. Fitzpatrick, designed an empowerment program for clinical nurses that helps them celebrate their contributions, to patients, their communities, and the world. She is the mother of six children and lives in Brecksville, Ohio, with her husband, Mark. Her favorite pastime is reading to her grandchildren.

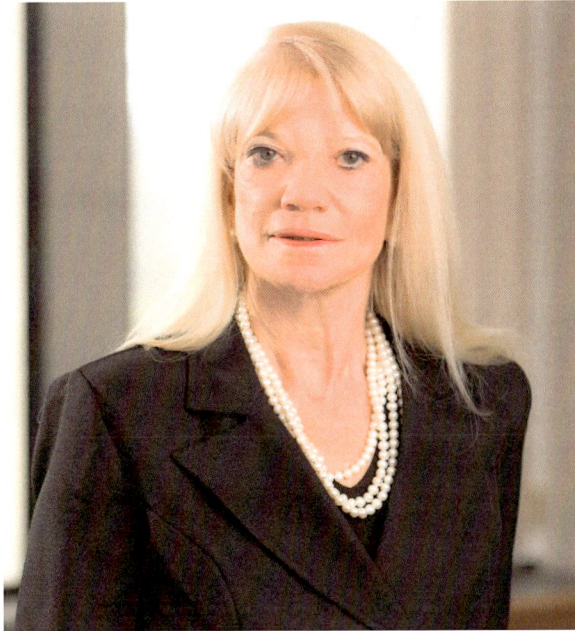

Joyce J. Fitzpatrick, PhD, MBA, RN, FAAN, FNAP, is Director of the Marian K. Shaughnessy Nurse Leadership Academy and Elizabeth Brooks Ford Professor of Nursing, Frances Payne Bolton School of Nursing, Case Western Reserve University (CWRU) in Cleveland, Ohio. She is an award-winning author with over 400 publications, including more than 80 books. She is a Living Legend in nursing. She has two daughters and three grandchildren, Penelope, Augustus, and Calliope.

CONTRIBUTORS

Joselyn Modic Banda received her bachelor's and master's degrees with Montessori credentials from Xavier University. She is Head of school and leads the primary classroom at a Montessori School in Fishers, Indiana. She and her husband, David, are the parents of two young daughters, Beatriz and Louise. She has introduced hundreds of children to the magic of reading and cultivated their imagination through stories.

Janna Draine Kinney received her BSN from Howard University and her M.Ed in Nursing from Drexel University. She is currently a nursing instructor at Case Western Reserve University in Cleveland, Ohio, where she lives with her husband and son.

Claire Modic is a Registered Nurse on a neurology/neurosurgery unit at a teaching hospital in Denver Colorado. She earned a BSN from Regis University in Denver, and a BS in Biology from Xavier University, Cincinnati, Ohio.

Nancy Busch Montgomery received her MFA from Ohio University. She is a teaching assistant at a grade school in Columbus, Ohio. She and her husband, Doug, are the parents of two grown sons.

Peter Stoffan is a Nurse Leader and trained singer/actor. He loves singing for his patients and team members whenever possible. He received his education from New York University and Indiana University. He currently resides in the Greater New York City area.

www.ingramcontent.com/pod-product-compliance
Lightning Source LLC
Chambersburg PA
CBRC090923150426
42812CB00061B/2669